Keto Diet for Beginners 2020

The Complete Guide to Lose Weight and Burn Fat Quickly and Easily on the Ketogenic Diet

By Meredith Blackmon

Table Of Contents

INTRODUCTION

The need to be slim or slender as a fashion norm is not new and has been further fueled by societal norms of what is acceptable and what is not. The fashion industry as always supported a certain look but being body conscious has increased among many due to the advent of social media. With many apps that are available for one to take pictures and share them with others, there is this increase to have the perfect image. One aspect of this image is to be of the perfect weight.

But being concerned about one's look is not a new ideology. Many have sought ways over the years to lose weight and keep it off, even though at times their desires are unrealistic. Some have sought medical assistance in reaching their desired look and weight. This may be in the form of evasive measures (surgeries), where they are nipped and tucked, and the fat sucked out of the body or even the stomach size decreased. There are other non-evasive methods (laser treatment, gastric balloons, etc.) that are being promoted as well. Others have sought to reduce their weight through natural means and thus, they adhere to specific dietary plans.

Yet with the health craze that has been developing over the years, people are not only concerned with their looks but their overall health and wellbeing. This means that they are more conscious of what they eat and are now more aware of how their diets may affect their quality of life and longevity. Over the years, various diets have been used to help people lose weight and maintain a healthy lifestyle. Diets such as the Atkins diet, the Paleo diet, and even the Sirtfood diet have proposed that following them will allow people to achieve the best quality of life from the foods that they eat.

Like other diets, the keto diet is based on scientific principles that guide its followers of the best foods to eat and in what quantity to get the best results. Within this book, you are going to be introduced to what the keto diet is – detailing how the understanding of the body and its functions supports the dietary plan. There will also be an examination of the benefits of following the diet and also side effects that may be encountered when they have started the process of using the diet to lose weight. The book also delves into some questions that are frequently asked by those who wish to follow the ketogenic lifestyle and a breakdown of the macronutrients within its plan. In addition, meal planning will be discussed and samples of recipes for breakfast, lunch, snacks, and desserts will be provided as a guide for those who wish to adhere to the keto diet.

There will be information presented on how you can use exercise alongside the diet to enhance your weight loss and basically improve your overall health. The final chapter will detail evidence of how following the keto diet can help persons who are suffering from certain ailments.

So, if you are new to the keto diet, this guide will help you in understanding what it is, the benefits that you can gain through its use and most importantly, understanding how you can apply the keto diet to your current lifestyle. No matter the reason for you desiring to adhere to a dietary plan, with this simplistically written and easy to understand guide, you are able to follow the principles provided so that you can lose weight and live a healthy and happy life.

CHAPTER ONE – THE BASICS

Common questions asked about the keto diet

So, before we get into the nitty-gritty of the diet, let's examine some frequently asked questions that people have about this diet. When embarking on this new adventure of following a keto diet, there may be some questions that you may have and need answers for. Though provided with brief answers here, as you read this guide you will delve into different aspects of the keto diet and will be able to gain a better understanding of its key guidelines.

1. How much weight will I lose?

The real answer to this question is based entirely on an individual – it is up to you! If you add an exercise regimen to the diet, then the rate of your weight loss will increase. When you remove items that may stall your progress, you will be able to progress further. These "stall" items include artificial sweeteners, dairy, wheat products and its by-product (wheat gluten, wheat flours, etc.).

However, what you will initially lose is water weight. One effect of ketosis is diuretic and so you will lose some pounds in the first couple of days. This is not fat loss though, but it is indicative that your body is starting to adjust and is entering the fat-burning phase.

You should note that stress, lack of sleep, exercise, alcohol intake and hormonal changes may slow down your weight loss. Losing weight is not a linear process and you will have fluctuations in your weight based on your daily intake of food or activities. If your weight loss slows down, you may consider rechecking your macros intake, drinking more water or electrolytes supplements or even reduce the amount of milk you consume.

On average, if you follow the keto diet you may lose between 1 to 2 pounds weekly, but this loss is not one that may happen consistently. It is best to take measurements as well to better help you track your weight loss for you may see a difference in the clothing size you wear and not necessarily weight reduction. If you see no changes after five weeks, it may be time to choose another diet plan.

2. How should I track my carb intake?

There are quite a number of free mobile apps that can be used to track your carb intake. One such example is MyFitnessPal. Even though you cannot track net carbs, you can track your overall carbohydrate and even dietary fiber intake. Another app is FatSecret.

3. What if I ate something that was forbidden on the diet?

Yes, you have deviated from your plan, but keep calm. Your weight may go up slightly as you regain some water weight. However, when you begin to get back on track, that weight will disappear. So, if your weight fluctuates, don't worry. It is due to our body gaining and losing water weight. You just need to stay vigilant and avoid the food items that take you from the stage of ketosis.

4. I don't like meat, eggs, dairy or a few other food items, can I still do a ketogenic diet?

The keto diet can still be followed if you do not consume certain types of foods. Following the keto diet is simply following the basic rules as discussed before. So, as long as you are low on carb, are consuming a moderate amount of protein a high level of fats, and all of this fits into your daily macros and calorie intake, then you should be fine.

Some users of the diet may drink coffee with butter and eat a lot of meat. For vegetarians, they may intake their proteins and fats in other ways. There are many options out there and so you can still follow the keto diet even if you have dietary restrictions.

5. What can I do after I have reached my target weight?

So, you may reach your desired weight goal, now what? Even when your goal is met, you can still adhere to the principles of the keto diet. Some people still do because it makes them feel better. However, note that if your old eating habits return, you will regain the weight. Even if you monitor your intake, you may still experience slight weight gain because of the refilling of your glycogen stores.

6. What is keto-adaptation? How long does it take to adapt?

Keto adaptation, also known as fat-adaption refers to the process of ketosis in which the body is able to make that switch from using glucose (sugar and carbohydrates) as the main source of energy, to the use of fat that has been stored in the body and that which is consumed through foods. When your body makes this switch varies for each individual and but may begin after just a few days after starting the diet. You are able to know by experiencing certain side effects which will be discussed later on in this guide. Sometimes within one to two weeks, people state they feel the positive effects the diet is having on their health and weight loss goals.

7. As my body begins to adapt to the keto diet, what changes are expected?

Though symptoms of starting the keto diet have been explained above, it should be reiterated that during the keto-adaptation process, there are some common side effects that some people may experience. These are related to what is called the "keto flu." There are also so uncommon ones that only a few people may experience. These symptoms are experienced because of the changes taking place in the body. The body is now switching to fat-burning mode and so these are going to be the changes that your body will experience when it stops using carbohydrates as the main source of energy. Sometimes the symptoms are compared to the withdrawal symptoms of addicts. In fact, your body was previously addicted to sugars and carbohydrates. So, what are the common symptoms experienced? Persons who experience the keto flu will normally feel sleepy, have aches and pains, feel the urge to vomit, are at times start feeling irritable or agitated and dizzy. For some, the symptoms will also include the soreness of the muscles, cramping and even stomach aches.

8. How long do the effects of the "keto flu" last?

As noted, the keto flu is a temporary effect and usually lasts for less than a week. Also, remember that not everyone experiences these symptoms. However, if you experience these symptoms, here are some suggestions that can aid in alleviating them:

• You will need to increase the electrolytes in your body. However, try to avoid manufactured electrolyte drinks as these will include added sugars.

• Remember to drink at up to a gallon of water each day.

• Don't limit your fat consumption. Eat more healthy fats.

• Purchase and take daily doses of ketone salts

• Become more physically active. Introduce working out/exercise to your lifestyle.

• Sleep at least eight hours per day. Rest is very important.

9. Is the keto diet safe? How long can I follow such a plan?

Like any other diet, the length of time you adhere to the rules is dependent on a person's preference and health goals. Or it may be that your doctor has recommended a specific time period for you to be on the ketogenic diet. There are many cultures and people who have practiced the diet for extended periods of time and have not experienced any negative effects.

10. Since I am eating more fats, will it raise my cholesterol levels?

As you continue to read this chapter, you will begin to realize that the myth that cholesterol is bad is not true. In fact, eating food with cholesterol actually barely increases cholesterol levels in the body. The truth is that what is harmful is high levels of triglycerides in the blood. This is a major risk factor for heart disease. These triglycerides in the blood are related to the consumption of a diet with high carbohydrate intake. It is when on the keto diet you are able to reduce the number of triglycerides in the blood. It would be best to visit your health care provider when following the keto diet to ensure that they are able to monitor blood cholesterol levels and they are within normal limits.

Historical Perspective

Like many diets that are being used today, the ketogenic diet is not one that is new to the health scene. The diet has been used over the years but initially gained most of its recognition through the effects experienced by its followers. The diet has been seen as a way to treat epilepsy. The idea is a person with epilepsy fasts or stops eating food, then the seizures that they will experience would stop over time. This was confirmed based on the results of a study conducted in France in 1910 which showed that fasting was a treatment for epilepsy. Further studies also showed that not only did the seizures stop but it was also seen that there was some improvement in mental activity when the body was being starved. However, it is impossible for someone to fast indefinitely unless they desire to die. Therefore, other means were needed to be used to help patients with epilepsy.

Through the research of Dr. Wilder of the Mayo Clinic in 1921, where he used the ketogenic diet to help treat people who suffered from the debilitating effect of the ailment, we can see how it is beneficial to our health. He also used the diet to prolong ketosis in diabetic patients. It was around the same time that when doctors from the Johns Hopkins Department of Pediatrics, Drs Howland and Gamble noticed that a diet which consisted of "prayer and a water" and basic starvation up to four weeks aided in the reduction of seizures in a nephew of one of their colleagues. Additional studies on the ketogenic diet have been conducted by Drs Lennox and Cobb at Harvard University.

Another doctor of the Mayo Clinic, Dr. Peterman, began using the diet regularly by 1924 and had achieved some level of success. In the 1930s, the diet became widely used as a form of treatment for epilepsy. After World War II ended, a doctor from Johns Hopkins University conducted a study with over 1,000 participants and found that the ketogenic diet was effective in controlling seizures. When more effective medications were being introduced to treat the symptoms of epilepsy, interest in the ketogenic diet declined.

A new thrust was seen in the 1980s and this interest in the diet was further developed when Dr. John Freeman at Johns Hopkins University revealed findings for a study conducted in 1992. The findings saw that the diet helped 30% of the children, who participated in the study, control seizures hey could not have previously controlled. In fact, due to its success, the parents of one of the children, Charlie Abrahams, helped to establish the Charlie foundation as a sign of their gratitude. It is through this foundation that the diet was widely spread and became more popular through a free videotape created for distribution.

Basics of the keto diet

The crux of a keto diet is the restriction of the consumption of carbohydrates (or carbs). Carbohydrates are normally found in foods such as pasta and bread and other sugary foods. It is not that no carbohydrates will not be consumed as it is needed in our diet, but the intake will be limited. Also known as a low-carb/high-fat (LCHF) of a strict low-carb diet, the keto diet is tailored so that you eat a lower percentage of carbohydrates and a higher percentage of fat.

For a long time, it has been ingrained in us the consumption of fat should be avoided. However, at the same time, many products being stated as being "low-fat" are those that have been laced with sugar to help to alleviate the change in the flavor profile when fat has been reduced. So, instead of helping to alleviate the obesity endemic, it propelled it further.

There are numerous researches today that counters the belief that fat is not good. These studies state that "good" fats which are natural do not need to be avoided. It is believed that heavy fat in our diets is healthy and instead one should aim to reduce the levels of sugar and starches within our diet.

Therefore, this makes it possible for us to eat foods that we love and still be able to lose weight.

Sugar and starches affect our blood sugar level. When we avoid or limit the consumption of foods that contain them, our blood sugar level stabilizes and therefore insulin, the hormones which help to store fats in our bodies, levels will drop. In turn, you will feel more satiated and it increases the fat burning mechanisms in our bodies – helping us to eat less and lose weight.

Another name for the keto diet is ketogenic diet. Eating a diet high in carbohydrates will cause your body to produce glucose and insulin. But if you adhere to the principles of the keto diet, your body will produce ketones that can be used as energy. These ketones are created in the liver.

Here are some facts related to the keto diet:

1. The main source of stored energy that the body will use is glucose. It is mostly used because it can easily be converted by the body to be used as energy.

2. In order for the body to process insulin, glucose is needed. As noted, the body will choose to use glucose first, so fats are then stored because they are not needed.

3. On a high carbohydrate diet, the body will use the glucose from the foods eaten as the

main source of energy. If the intake of carbohydrates is lowered, then the body will go into ketosis.

What is Ketosis?

When we lessen the amount of food we consume, our bodies begin to naturally go into a state where their aim is to survive. It is within this state that ketones are produced. These ketones are responsible for breaking down the fats in our liver. The overall goal for the state of ketosis is for our body to go into a metabolic state. This state is only reached through the reduction of carbohydrates and not the limitation of calories. Also, it should be noted that due to the adaptive nature of our bodies, we are able to use ketones as the main source of energy if we consume fats with fewer carbohydrates. All parts of our bodies – including the brain and organs will be dependent on ketones for energy to perform their functions. What science recognizes is the fact that ketone is a better source of energy because it is more stable than the use of glucose which we consume through our carbohydrate intake. In eating a diet that is low in carbohydrates, you are to eat more proteins and healthy fats. The proteins should be of high-quality (unprocessed) and only "good" or healthy fats should be consumed.

Placing your body in the state of ketosis will allow us to achieve optimal health – weight loss and an increase in our mental and physical performance.

Recent studies have noted that the keto diet reduces the risk of developing lifestyle-related diseases such as diabetes, heart disease, stroke, and other diseases such as Alzheimer's and epilepsy.

For your body to enter the state of ketosis, you should have reduced your carbohydrate intake from a minimum of three (3) days to a week. The use of fats instead of carbohydrates for energy is not only from the fats that you eat but also from the fat stored in your body. To know if one has reached into the state of ketosis, checks can be made when the level of ketones can be measured through blood or urine samples. Checking the levels can help you to ensure that you are always in a state of ketosis throughout adhering to the diet.

How Does the Keto Diet Work?

Any diet that puts your body in the state of ketosis, so that your body is able to burn fat that is either consumed or already stored in the body, is called a ketogenic diet. Eating a high carb diet in today's society is becoming the norm. Note that many fast-food restaurants serve foods with high carbohydrate levels (burgers, pizzas, fries, etc.). In eating a high carb diet, your body uses glucose as the main source of energy. Though helpful to our bodies by providing it with energy, there are negative effects of having high levels of glucose in the bloodstream.

When we consume foods with sugar (glucose), the body converts it to glycogen and then stores it. Only

2,000 calories of glucose energy can be stored in the body at any given time. Whenever this storage is depleted, you begin to lose energy and experience the effects of "bonking" and your body begins to crave sugar to increase your energy levels. Note that excess sugar in the bloodstream increases insulin levels. It is insulin that determines if glucose is stored or if it is used. Insulin also indicates to the body that glucose should be stored in the liver by converting it into fat. Sugar from fruits (fructose) and those used for sweetening are not used as energy but are stored in the body as fat.

If you have an excess of glucose in the blood, you are at a higher risk of developing Type 2 diabetes. If this disease is not monitored and healthy lifestyle choices made, then it may progressively become worse and may lead to death or poor quality of life. Note that Type 2 diabetes is an irreversible lifestyle disease.

However, if you limit your intake of carbohydrates and consume healthy proteins and fats, insulin levels will decrease. This decline of insulin in the blood is a result of there being less glucose to be used. If the insulin level within your blood is low, then the fat that was previously stored in the liver for energy can be used as fuel/energy. This fat burning leads to the development of ketones in the body.

When you no longer consume the massive amounts of carbohydrates that are found in typical meals and you then eat more proteins and good fats, then there will be a decline in insulin levels. This is due to the fact that there will be limited glucose for the body to use as fuel. As noted, it Is when there is a decline in insulin levels then the fat that is stored in your liver or the fat that you eat can be burned. This is not possible unless your insulin levels are low.

When fat is burned, the ketones are created. Ketones are fatty acids that are used by most cells in the body, which can be used as fuel. Probably you believe that it is something that only a few people are capable of achieving. However, we all are capable of going into a state of ketosis. Scientists believe that over 180,000 years ago, human beings were naturally in the state of ketosis most of the time. This was possible due to their diet. They ate mostly animal protein and fat – at times they received nutrients from plants, nuts and fruits.

However, it should be known that not because the body is in a state of ketosis, it is able to convert fat into fuel efficiently. How so, you may ask. The process of your body going into the state of ketosis fully takes from three to eight weeks. It is in this time that your body becomes "fat-adapted" and "forgets" how to properly process glucose but is able to process fat and ketones effectively. At the time that you are fully "fat-adapted," you will feel energized as if you have a never-ending source of vitality. It is almost as if you could do a marathon and never get tired. When your body becomes the main source of energy, it does not need to be replenished with food.

In addition, it is expected that your cravings and hunger will diminish. If you do not consume carbs then you will not desire them. It is as if the more you are well adapted into the state of ketosis, the more you are able to avoid eating "carbage." It is believed that you will quickly lose weight and return to a healthy body weight.

If you are not committed to the keto diet, then it will not work for you. Cheating and consuming carbs will ruin all the progress that you have made. Therefore, it is suggested that you discard all the foods that are unhealthy before you begin the diet. Even though these foods were considered, you will not miss them because, with the keto diet, there are still some great food options available. We know that it will take much willpower to get started but once you experience the benefits of this diet, you will not want to revert to your old lifestyle.

Why We Get Fat?

The horrid word leptin has been circulating on the scientific scene over the last decade. This newly discovered hormone is said to play a great role in weight regulation in our bodies. Leptins are found in our fat cells and their main function is to communicate with the brain that you are feeling full – satiated. However, for many people, there are issues with this communication. Why? Because we have become leptin resistant. It has recently been discovered that leptin in our bodies is not functioning well because of insulin.

Insulin is the hormone that is wreaking havoc in our bodies. If they are not functioning well, then other hormones and bodily functions will not work effectively. We discussed before that insulin helps to convert sugar in our blood to body fat which is for the body a safe place to store extra calories you consume. For example, if a diabetic has high blood sugar (over the 100-limit) and they take a shot of insulin, their blood sugar level would decrease. Where did that excess sugar go? It was stored as energy in our fat cells by the hormone. High blood sugar is detrimental to our health as well. It can lead to Type 2 diabetes , kidney failure, fatty liver, and even cancer. It is high insulin levels in our bodies that cause fats to be stored in our bodies instead of calories being burned.

Then it is fair to ask why the leptin that is stored in our fat is unable to indicate to our brains that we are full? It is the insulin that blocks the leptin receptors from communicating that to the brain. It is having the feeling of still feeling hungry or unsatisfied even when the stomach is full. So, you just had that burger, fries and soda. But what you should know is that foods such as these have carbohydrates which cause your blood sugar level to rise, and your pancreas will secrete more insulin. As you get older, the insulin produced by your body becomes less effective. At this point in time, it will take fat to the cells, but the cells will refuse it and more insulin is required to do the job. Eventually, we will develop insulin resistance and then Type 2 diabetes.

So, how do we alleviate the problem we have discussed above? It's simple; we should reduce the amount of insulin that our pancreas secretes. This cannot be done by eating less and exercising more. We will need to also reduce the number of carbohydrates we consume.

When you follow a keto diet for just a few days, you will lose the desire to consume sugars and starches and you will feel so much better. You will also feel the desire to eat less because the leptin is able to do its job – not being hindered by the insulin.

High Fat Consumption: healthy or unhealthy?

The keto diet advises that we get most of our macronutrients from fat. This was something that was previously frowned upon and deemed unhealthy. Is it? No, it is not if you are consuming saturated fats. As previously discussed, eating a low-fat diet does not help to make you healthier. Studies have shown that such a diet has actually increased the likelihood of obesity and diabetes.

The belief that fat consumption is dangerous was purported by Ancel Keys. He hypothesized that eating fats will result in heart disease. Though his theory is easy to understand – just like how sugar ends up in or blood, so will fat – it was completely wrong. The liver actually makes the fat that is found in the blood and it is a diet with high sugar consumption that actually leads to the increased levels of fat being circulated in our blood. These fats are called triglycerides.

However, it was through effective persuasion methods that he was able to demonstrate these now refuted ideas. In his studies, he used data collected from countries that suggested that there is a correlation between saturated fat and heart disease. If data from some countries did not support this idea, they were known as paradoxes. One such is data from France. The "French paradox" is that even though the French ate a high level of saturated fats, they had the lowest rates of heart disease. This was also true for the Swiss and the Russian Mortality Paradox – where they eat the highest concentration of fats but have the lowest deaths due to heart disease. The lifestyle of the Inuit or "Eskimos" of the Artic also contradicts the views of Keys. They not only consume fish, seal and whale meat, but they even eat blubber. The lean meats are mostly fed to the dogs. Yet they have a low rate of heart disease.

Even though there was evidence to prove that Keys' theory was wrong, it was greatly supported by the USDA and adopted into dietary guidelines that we still use today. For eating a keto diet rich in fats, it actually allows our body to burn the fat for fuel. Even though it sounds unhealthy to eat a cheeseburger with extra cheese, bacon and mayo, it is actually healthy if you remove the buns.

Ketones

We previously defined what is ketosis. But let us now delve further into how it is created and the types that our body has.

Our body produces ketones because of the process of the liver breaking down some of the fats in our body for fuel. When our body processes fats like this, we are said to be in a state of ketosis. Our body then produces three types of ketones: acetone, acetoacetate, and beta-hydroxybuterate acid.

As we enter into the state of ketosis, our body initially produces acetoacetate (sometimes known as pees tick ketone). This is the ketone that is easily measured through our urine. Our body will convert a portion into acetones (breath ketone and then and enzymatically converted it into the ketone which the brain normally uses for energy called beta-hydroxybuterate. As our bodies adapt to the diet, we are able to efficiently create beta-hydroxybutyrate dehydrogenase. It is the creation of acetone that makes those following the diet develop bad breath and sometimes body odor. But these effects diminish after some time.

Just as how our body cells could use glucose, so can they use ketones directly. However, there are a few cell types (red blood cells, cells that make up the eye and parts of your brain) that require the use of glucose. Not to worry though. Your liver actually has a built-in glucose generator that is able to create glucose from the protein we ingest through the process of gluconeogenesis (gluco = sugar, neo = new, genesis = create). Therefore, your liver is able to create enough "new sugar: for those vital cells to use. This isn't something new but a process that existed for a long time or we were able to live without carbs for such a long time.

Ketoacidosis

Is it possible for the state of ketosis to be harmful? This is a yes, but only if things are taken to the extreme. When this happens, your body goes into the state of ketoacidosis because your ketone levels are too high, and your blood begins to become acidic. At this stage, you are at an increased risk of developing Type 1 diabetes. However, if you have a properly functioning pancreas, it is highly unlikely for you to go into this stage.

If you already have Type 1 diabetes, it is advised that you do not attempt this diet without proper supervision and guidance from a healthcare professional. But those with Type 2 diabetes or are prediabetic should be safe to follow the keto diet.

Testing for Ketones

One most common way to attempt to test if your body is in a state of ketosis is to use what are called pee strips. However, the pee strips only test for acetoacetate and this is only an indication of the ketones that are wasted. As you become more "fat adapted" then these levels will decrease, and the indication of the strips will become lighter as your body will be using more ketones. Therefore, the best way to check for ketones is through a breath test such as the breath meters such as the Ketonic or to do a blood test through the use of products such as the Freestyle Precision Neo glucometer.

Still, there are numerous other ways you can know if your body is in the state of ketosis. These include signs and symptoms from your body which let you know that you are on the right track, such as:

- Frequent urination. Since the diet is a natural diuretic, you may produce more urine and you may need to use the bathroom more. This is most common in those beginning the diet because of the increase in acetoacetate in their bodies.

- Increased thirst and dry mouth. Because you are urinating frequently, you begin to experience an increased desire for fluid intake and the feeling that the mouth is dry. Ensure to replace the fluids you are losing by drinking a lot of water and replenish the electrolytes (salt, potassium, magnesium) lost.

- Bad breath. We previously discussed that this is caused by the production of acetones. Your breath may have the smell that is similar to overripe fruits or even nail polish remover. This effect is temporary.

- Reduced hunger and increased energy. After the effects of the "keto flu" where you feel lethargic and tired, you will experience a lower appetite and increased energy levels (physically and mentally).

Basic ketogenic meals

We have discussed macronutrients, and this is great information, but let's delve into what a keto diet meal actually looks like. In such a meal, you will have only 10% of calories coming from leafy greens, non-starchy vegetable or any other healthy carbohydrates. You may also consume small amounts of legumes and berries. For proteins that make up 20% of the calories you consume daily, they will be derived from omega-3-rich fish and grass-fed animal protein. Finally, 70% of calories eaten are from high-quality fats such as avocado, unsaturated and medium-chain triglyceride oils, nuts and seeds, and coconut.

Therefore, the ratio of 10:20:70 is the typical guideline for each person. However, your doctor may recommend varying percentages based on your levels of physical activity and personal health goals.

Ketogenic Diets for fat and muscle gains

If you are desirous of building muscles, this section is a good read. You may be asking if carbohydrates are necessary to build muscle. They are not needed for that. Therefore, a keto diet is an excellent way for you to build muscle mass. What is most important is the intake of protein. If you wish to gain muscle mass, then 1.0 to 1.2 grams of protein by lean pound is needed daily.

If you are desirous of building body fat, then there are types of ketogenic diets that you can try:

■ Standard Ketogenic Diet (SKD): the standard keto diet.

■ Targeted Ketogenic Diet (TKD): you will follow the regular principles of consuming a SKD but only consuming a small amount of fast-digesting carbs before a workout.

■ Cyclical Ketogenic Diet (CKD): for bodybuilders, you will consume more carbs on that day to resupply glycogen stores.

Recently, other types of keto diets have pop up. These are known as the lay keto or the dirty keto. As the name lazy suggests, there is no real monitoring of the carb intake even though the followers of this diet try to have between 20 to 50 grams of carbs each day. The idea of the dirty keto is that the same levels of macronutrients daily are adhered to, but the followers take these from any source – it doesn't matter where they come from, as long as the required amounts are consumed.

These versions are not long-lasting, and they negatively affect your overall health and wellbeing. Since good habits are not being formed, persons following these variations can easily slip back into their normal eating patterns. However, there are numerous people who have posted on websites saying that these versions have actually helped them lose weight.

Benefits of a Ketogenic Diet

Many people will follow the diet for the most common effect, which is weight loss and increased energy. However, this and other benefits will be discussed below.

Weight Loss

Since the diet results in the body using body fat for energy, there will be evident weight loss benefits. With the keto diet, our fat-storing hormone, insulin, will turn our bodies into a lean, mean, fat-burning machine. The weight loss experienced from the ketogenic diet is greater in comparison to low-fat and high- carb diets in the long term. Some people report that including MCT oil and drinking coffee in the morning will increase ketone production and ultimately fat loss.

Control Blood Sugar

When you no longer ingest the number of sugars and carbohydrates that you used to, your blood sugar levels will lower and be maintained at a healthy level. Research has provided evidence that following the keto diet will manage and prevent diabetes. This possibility is even greater than following a low-calorie diet. Even if you are pre-diabetic or have Type 2 diabetes, the keto diet is still beneficial to your health.

Mental Focus

If you desire to increase your mental performance, the keto diet is one that is most beneficial. Just as how ketones are created when the fats in our body are used. These ketones actually are a great source of energy for the brain. Because a low-carb diet will result in big spikes in blood sugar, you can have improved focus and concentration. In addition, research also shows the benefits of increased fat consumption also include improved focus and concentration and fatty acids will improve brain function.

Hunger

Consumption of too many carbs and sugars make you crave them even more. In following the keto diet, you will have more energy, but the consumption of fat will leave you feeling satiated (full) for longer and therefore, you will ultimately eat less. This is a great recipe for more weight loss.

Epilepsy

Did you know that the keto diet has been used to treat people with epilepsy since the 1900s? This is true and it is able to treat it successfully. It is even used today to aid children with uncontrolled epilepsy. The diet will allow patients with the ailment to start using fewer medications. Recent research has shown that the keto diet can help adults with epilepsy as well.

Cholesterol and Blood Pressure

For persons who have high triglyceride and cholesterol levels that can lead to arterial buildup, they will have such levels reduced when they are on a keto diet. Being a low carb/high-fat diet, it will increase HDL and decrease LDL particle concentration when compared to low-fat diets.

The diet will also result in properly controlled and maintained healthy blood pressure levels. Since there is a correlation to elevated blood pressure levels and obesity, there will be a decrease in those levels, and you lose weight.

Insulin Resistance

If levels of insulin are not properly managed, then this will result in insulin resistance and then further to Type 2 diabetes. The keto diet will result in lowered insulin levels into ranges that are healthy. The keto diet is especially beneficial to those who are athletic because they benefit from greater insulin usage through eating foods high in omega-3 fatty acids.

Acne

There are great skin benefits to be experienced when you follow the keto diet. One study shows that there will be fewer occurrences of lesions or even skin inflammation. In another study, there shows some possible correlation between a high-carb diet and increased acne. So, it is assumed that the fewer carbs one eats, is the fewer chances of developing acne. Also, it will be beneficial for you to reduce the intake of milk and just by using a strict skin cleaning routine.

How to Reach Ketosis

It is simple for one to reach the stage of ketosis. Here are some steps that are easy to follow:

1. Limit carbohydrate intake. Though most people focus on net carbs if you want the best results limit the intake of all carbs. It is recommended that you consume below 20g net carbs and below 35g total carbs per day.

2. Pay close attention to our protein intake. Though other diets (such as the Atkins diet) do not limit the proteins consumed, too much protein may slow or lower your level of ketosis. So, if you desire weight loss, it is best for you to consume high-quality protein (0.6g and 0.8g for each pound that you weigh). Use a keto calculator to help you know the correct amount.

3. Ensure that you drink a sufficient amount of water. Try drinking up to a gallon each day. Just stay hydrated and be consistent with the amount you drink. The consumption of water helps your body to regulate its functions and control your hunger.

4. Avoid having snacks. Snacks help to increase your insulin spikes which will negatively affect your weight loss plan.

5. Try fasting. When you fast, you are able to boost ketone levels throughout the day.

6. Exercise regularly. The benefits that can be derived from exercise are well-known facts but these increase when you are following a keto diet. So, even 20 to 30 minutes of exercise each day can help you to regulate weight loss and blood sugar levels.

7. Take supplements. Restrictions in the diet may lead to a shortage of supplements. So, take supplements such as daily vitamins. However, check the labels to ensure that these are made with keto-friendly ingredients.

Common Side Effects on a Keto Diet

Though there are many health benefits to be derived when following a keto diet, the diet also has its drawbacks. Below are the most frequently experienced side effects faced by those who have just begun to adhere to the rules of the diet. Note that with the reduction of carbohydrates in the diet most side effects will be related to either dehydration or because of the lack of micronutrients (vitamins) in the body due to the restrictions of food to be consumed. Therefore, ensure that you are drinking sufficient amounts of water daily (again, up to a gallon a day is recommended as opposed to the generally suggested 6-8 glasses). It is also important that based on the acceptable foods in the diet, you should consume foods rich in micronutrients (vitamins), and these can also be consumed by taking supplemental multivitamins and essential minerals daily.

Cramps

You are more than likely to experience leg cramps when starting the diet. These cramps normally occur in the morning or at night. However, they do not majorly affect you. These cramps are indicative of a lack of necessary minerals in the body, most notably magnesium. Drinking a lot of water as well as including some salt in your diet may help to alleviate this symptom. You may also consider to orally ingest magnesium supplements.

Constipation

Because of the risk of dehydration, you may also experience constipation. Drinking more water may aid in alleviating this issue. To alleviate this, please follow the suggestion and drink close to a gallon of water each day; I can't stress this enough. Dehydration is by far the most common cause of constipation you may experience initially on the keto diet. Increasing your fiber intake is also a possible solution. Therefore, consume vegetables that are high in fiber. Vegetables which are good sources of fiber are ones that are non-starchy. If the problem persists, you may consider taking fiber powders or even in ingesting a probiotic.

Heart Palpitations

At the beginning of the diet, you may feel your heart beating faster and harder. This is known as heart palpitations. If you experience this, do not worry; it is a pretty standard side effect. Again, remedy this by increasing your water intake and ensure that you are eating enough salt. Normally, if you do as suggested, the problem will cease to exist, immediately. However, you may also consider taking a potassium supplement daily.

Reduced Physical Performance

When beginning the keto diet, you may not have the levels of energy that you usually have. However, this will not persist as your body is beginning to adapt to using fat instead of glucose as an energy source. After your body as transitioned into this change, your energy level, strength and endurance will return to its normal level. If the problem persists, consider having some carbohydrates before you work out.

Other Side Effects

There are some other side effects that are not as common as those discussed above. These include:

Breastfeeding

There may be some effects related to beginning the keto diet when breastfeeding, though there are no thorough studies that may confirm this. For now, one can assume that beginning the keto diet may be a safe venture when breastfeeding.

However, it is recommended that you add 30-50g extra carbs from fruit which will help your body to produce milk. Since the macronutrients and calories in your body affect milk production, you may add in extra calories from healthy food sources. 300 to 500 extra calories can provide extra fat necessary for milk production. It is best to seek advice from a health professional before beginning this diet.

Hair Loss

Losing hair is another least common side effect of adhering to the restrictions of the ketogenic diet. You may lose hair between the first five months of starting this diet, however, this is temporary. Therefore, do not worry; continue to take your multivitamins and continue with the process. Though this is an uncommon symptom, if it persists, check to ensure that you are not eating too few calories and you are getting enough rest. It is recommended that you sleep up to eight (8) hours each night.

Increased Cholesterol

Increased cholesterol in your bloodstream is normally a good thing, especially when related to the increase in good cholesterol (HDL). Studies noted that there may be an increase in cholesterol levels when following the keto diet. With the increase in the good cholesterols in your bloodstream, you have a lowered risk of heart disease. Even if you see an increase in triglyceride, this is a common side effect of people who are losing weight. This will be reduced when weight loss is normalized.

Only a few people experience raised LDL cholesterol. Though it is harder to detect, this is common and not harmful. It only becomes harmful when there is a greater level of LDL than the normal level for a healthy diet.

Gallstones

Only a small percentage of research on the keto diet show that people who have been afflicted with gallstones have the such reduced or diminished when on the keto diet. A question of importance is: is it safe to follow the keto diet if one has their gallbladder removed? Yes, it is okay and will not cause any adverse effects.

It is suggested that fat intake should be increased gradually so that your body may become used to the change.

Indigestion

If you ever have issues with indigestion or heartburn, the keto diet is one that is very helpful to alleviate those ailments. However, some people may experience such when they are starting the diet. If you have experienced any of these symptoms, it is suggested that you limit your intake of fats and gradually increase each day over a two weeks period.

Keto Rash

Itching is another uncommon issue that some people may face when beginning the keto diet. Though there is no scientific evidence to explain why some people may have this experience, there are some written experiences of such. Some explain the itching as being a result of their sweat being laced with acetone (aby product of ketosis which also results in bad breath. Therefore, extra hygienic measures should be taken to alleviate sweat remaining on the body – by changing your clothes and showering often. It may also be suggested that you increase your carbs or make changes to your exercise routine.

Damage to the Heart

Some researchers have stated that the keto diet may cause some damage to the heart. They believe that this is because the diet normally focuses on gaining much of the daily recommended proteins and fat from animals. This they believe will have a negative effect on heart health as it can increase one's risk of cardiovascular disease or it may worsen it in cases where people have already been diagnosed with it.

In fact, it is believed that persons may be at a greater risk for hypertension, especially if they have a family with a history of this disease. Therefore, users are asked to be cautious when following this diet.

Saving Money and Budgeting

There are some who believe that following the keto diet is an expensive venture. Even though purchasing carbohydrate filled foods may be a cheaper option, the diet is not as expensive as people may think.

You may use the following tips to help you save money while following the diet. It is just as simple as using a budget to help you save money.

Try to find deals. Finding a sale or using a coupon to purchase keto-friendly foods is a win-win. These coupons can be typically found in magazines and newspapers. In-store coupons and store discounts may also help to reduce your shopping bill.

Buy and cook in bulk. Some of us do not like to spend a lot of time in the kitchen or even shopping. Therefore, if you can buy foods in bulk (for example, from wholesalers) you can reduce your cost per pound significantly. You can also prepare foods in bulk for storage and use leftovers. Doing such will decrease the amount of time spent in the kitchen.

Cook your own food. Due to convenience, we may be lured to purchase foods that are pre-made or pre-cooked. These tend to be more expensive. However, it is best to cook your own foods from natural ingredients. It is cheaper and it is a healthier option. So, prepare your vegetables instead of buying pre-cut ones and use cheaper cuts of meat (chuck roast) to make your stews.

Basic Takeaways

The overall idea of the keto diet is that eating high levels of fat with proteins and lessening our carbohydrate intake can positively impact our overall health. This means that your cholesterol will be lowered, you will lose and maintain a healthy body weight and blood sugar levels. You may also see an increase in your energy levels and will see yourself experiencing a good mood more.

The diet may be a bit hard to follow in the beginning, but it becomes easier over time. Continue to stay on track and you will see how the diet is good in helping you keep a healthy lifestyle. So, it is advised that you:

– Keep your meal plans simple and stay true to the rules of the diet.

- Limit the number of carbs you consume, especially in the first month. You will see better results.

- While cutting excess sweets, you should also avoid the use of artificial sweeteners. These include those found in diet sodas. When you do so, your sugar cravings will decrease.

- Drink a lot of water and supplement electrolytes.

- Take your multivitamins

- Try by all means to consume the daily recommended amount of sodium.

- Track what you eat. Sometimes carbs are hidden, and you may over-consume them. When you keep track of what you consume, you are able to keep yourself accountable for the results.

CHAPTER TWO - CALORIES and MACRONUTRIENTS

What are calories?

When we eat, we consume calories. These are actually units of energy that is used by the body. When you read the nutritional content of a package and it states that the food contains 100 calories, it is actually stating that this is the amount of energy your body will receive if you eat it all. With any weight loss plan, the intake of calories will determine if you are successful or not. If you consume more calories than your body needs to function, then you will gain weight. Take for example consuming each day 2,000 calories but your body only requires 1,800 then you are consuming more than the body needs – resulting in weight gain over time. However, if you do light exercise and you burn 300 calories that you have increased the calories required by the body – resulting in a calorie deficit of 100 calories. Continuously consuming a deficit of calories will overtime lead to weight loss because your body will continue to use the stored energy sources in the body – fat. Therefore, it is advised that you maintain a balance with the macronutrients in your body daily so that it has all the energy it needs.

What Are Macronutrients?

The molecules in our bodies that are used to create the energy that we need are called macronutrients (otherwise known as macros). These are simply known as fats, proteins and carbohydrates. These are typically found in the foods that we eat and are measured in grams (g) on nutrition labels. Each gram of fat that you eat is equivalent to nine calories. Your body will gain four calories for every gram of protein that you eat. Also, for each gram of carbohydrate, your body receives four calories.

Net Carbs

The net carbs within most low-carb recipes are written displaying the macros. Net carbs are the carbs where dietary fiber and sugar alcohols are not added In the total calculation. These are indigestible by the body and so they are not counted towards the carb total. Sometimes dietary fiber may be listed as either soluble or insoluble.

How Much Should You Eat?

Now that you have an understanding of calories, macronutrients and net carb, it is now time to gain an understanding of how much is suitable to be eaten when following a keto diet. Fat consumption is very important in a keto diet, so about 65% - 75% of your daily recommended diet should be from fat. About 20% - 30% of your daily intake should be protein. This leaves only 5% of carbs to be consumed.

To determine how many calories and the macros you should be eating each day, you will need to use a keto calculator. These can be found for free online.

Keto calculator

Though keto calculators may differ in style, they all require that you submit basic information such as your weight, activity levels and goals. After inputting such data, it instantly provides you with the grams of fat, protein and carbs you should be eating daily.

CHAPTER THREE - NUTRITIONAL REVOLUTION

Carbs: What Exactly Are They?

It has been mentioned numerous times so far that the consumption of carbohydrates on a keto diet should be limited. To be able to avoid these foods, then you should know what they are. If you consume foods that contain starches, grains foods that are high in sugar, then you are consuming foods that are high in carbs. These will include foods such as bread, flour, rice, pasta, beans, potatoes, sugar, syrup, cereals, fruits, bagels and soda.

When we consume carbs and they are broken into glucose for energy, we should note that each carb may provide a spike that is faster or slower. The rate is dependent on if the carb is simple or complex.

With these spikes, insulin is released to combat it. However, with such constant release then or fat storage and insulin resistance increases, leading to prediabetes, metabolic syndrome and even Type 2 diabetes.

With the typical diet in the world today, laden with sugar, it is very easy for us to overconsume carbs. So, the cereal, pasta, burgers, French fries and large sodas, contribute to our carb intake. Research shows that almost 1 in 10 adults in the US have Type 2 diabetes and this is an increase of almost four times more than 30 years ago.

In addition, according to the 2014 report by the Centers for Diseases Control and Prevention (CDC), more than 1 in every 3 adults in the U.S. (86 million people) have prediabetes. With prediabetes blood, glucose is always high. Other than previously believed, fat isn't at fault and so the low-fat and fat-free, chemically-laden alternatives are not helping to reduce the ever-increasing rates of diabetes and heart disease.

Fat is No Longer the Bad Guy

Most fats are healthy and essential to our overall health and large amounts of carbohydrates are detrimental to it. With the change in the precious mindset, there is an increase in keto/low carb and similar dietary groups. These are seen as the beginning of a food revolution. People are finally beginning to see that it is the excess sugar and carbs that are actually the bad guys that cause harm to their health.

But isn't fat bad for you? The answer to this question is complex in nature. It is a fact that too much fat may cause arteriosclerosis (blockages of the blood vessels). With the blockage of our blood vessels, we are at greater risk of heart attacks or strokes. Yet we cannot downplay the nutritional roles that fat plays in our overall health. Even cholesterol, in controlled amounts, is necessary.

Foods to Enjoy

Being on the keto diet does not mean that eating will not be an enjoyable experience. You can still have foods that are appetizing and filling while still sticking to the keto influenced eating regime. We'll examine some of these food items below:

Note that it has been emphasized in this book that though it is encouraged that one eats vegetables, these should be non-starchy.

Non-starchy Vegetables

Serving size:

Leafy greens: Approximately 2–3 cups, raw

All others: 1/2 cup cooked or 1 cup raw

- **Celery and celery root**

- **Arugula**

- **Collard Greens**

- **Artichoke**

- **Asparagus**

- Radicchio

- Dandelion

- Bamboo shoots

- Bean sprouts

- Bitter melon

- Bottle gourd

- Endive

- Broccoli

- Brussels sprouts

- Swiss Chard

- Cabbage (bok choy, green, nappa, red, savoy)

- Cactus (nopales)

- Cauliflower

- Chayote (Cho-Cho)

- Cucumber

- Watercress

- Eggplant

- Green beans (string beans)

- Hearts of palm

- Jerusalem artichoke

- Jicama

- Kimchi

- Kohlrabi

- Leeks

- Different varieties of lettuce (Romaine, Iceberg, etc.)

- Water Chestnuts

- Mushrooms

- Onions (green, brown, red, scallions, shallot, spring, white, yellow)

- Sweet Peppers

- Okra

- Red Peppers

- Jalapenos

- Habaneros

- Different types of radishes

- Rutabaga

- Sauerkraut

- Sea plants (arame, dulse, kombu, kelp, nori)

- Sprouts

- Sugar snap peas, snow peas

- Summer squash (crookneck, delicata, yellow, spaghetti, zucchini, pattypan)

- Tomatoes

- Turnips

1 serving = approx. 25 calories

Macronutrients: carbs= 5 g, protein = 1-2 g, fats = 0 g

Dairy

Serving size:

- Kefir, plain: 1 cup

- Milk: 1 cup

- Yogurt, plain, full-fat/whole milk, Greek: 1/2 cup

1 serving = approx. 100-150 calories

Macronutrients: carbohydrates = 12 g, protein = 8 g, fat = 5-8 g

Note: Full-fat dairy products recommended

Protein

Serving size

Salmon

- Canned: 3 oz.

- Fresh: 3 oz.

- Bacon: 2 slices

- Beef – all cuts: 3 oz.

Cheeses

- Buffalo: 3 oz.

- Cottage: 3/4 cup

- Feta: 2 oz.

- Goat: 2 oz.

- Mozzarella: 2 oz. or 1/2 cup shredded

- Ricotta: 1/3 cup

- Chicken, white or dark meat: 3 oz.

- Turkey, white or dark meat: 3 oz.

- Venison: 3 oz.

- Cornish hen: 4 oz.

- Smoked Herring: 3 oz.

- Smoked Mackerel: 2 oz.

- Sardines (in water or oil): 3 oz.

- Trout: 4 oz.

- Tuna

  Canned, chunk light or solid light (in water or oil): 4 oz.

- Shellfish (crab, clams, lobster, mussels, oysters, scallops): 4–5 oz.

- Skipjack: 4 oz.

- Yellowtail: 4 oz.

- Lamb, leg, chop, or lean roast: 3 oz.

- Liver: 3 oz.

- Eggs, whole: 2

- Egg whites: 1 cup

- Elk: 3 oz.

- Sausage: the portion varies

- Pork, tenderloin: 3 oz.

1 serving = approx. 150 calories

Macronutrients: carbohydrates = 0 g, protein = 14-28 g, fat = 1-9 g

Oils and Fats

Serving size:

- Ghee/clarified butter: 1 tsp.

- Grapeseed oil: 1 tsp.

- High-oleic safflower oil: 1 tsp.

- High-oleic sunflower oil: 1 tsp.

- Avocado: 2 Tbsp.

- Avocado oil: 1 tsp.

- Butter: 1 tsp.

- Canola: 1 tsp.

- Cream: 1 tsp.

- Cream cheese: 1 Tbsp.

- Flaxseed oil: 1 tsp.

- powder: 1/2 Tbsp.

- Olive oil, extra virgin: 1 tsp.

- Olives: 8–10 medium

- Sesame oil: 1 tsp.

- Sour cream: 2 Tbsp.

- Mayonnaise, unsweetened (made with avocado, grapeseed, or olive oil): 1 Tbsp.

- Medium-chain triglyceride oil: 1 tsp.

- Medium-chain triglyceride

- Coconut milk, light, canned: 3 Tbsp; regular, canned: 1.5 Tbsp.

- Coconut oil: 1 tsp.

- Coconut spread: 1.5 tsp.

1 serving = approx. 45 calories

Macronutrients: carbohydrates = 0 g, protein = 0 g, fat = 5 g

Nuts and Seeds

Serving size:

Almonds: 6

Almond butter: 1½ tsp.

Brazil: 2

Cashews: 6

Cashew butter: 1½ tsp.

Chia seeds: 1 Tbsp.

Coconut, unsweetened, shredded: 1½ Tbsp.

Flaxseed, ground: 1½ Tbsp.

Hazelnuts: 5

Hemp seeds: 2 tsp.

Macadamia: 3

Pecans: 2

Pine nuts: 1 Tbsp.

Pistachios: 12

Pumpkin seeds: 1 Tbsp.

Sesame seeds: 1 Tbsp.

Soy nuts, roasted: 2 Tbsp.

Sunflower seeds: 1 Tbsp.

Tahini: 11/2 tsp.

Walnuts: 2

1 serving = approx. 45 calories

Macronutrients: carbohydrate = 0 g, protein = 1 g, fat = 5 g

Beverages

Unlimited servings/day:

Coffee

Green tea (unsweetened)

Noncaffeinated herbal teas (mint, chamomile, hibiscus, etc.)

Bottled or Carbonated Mineral water

Filtered Water

Condiments/Herbs and Spices

Unlimited servings/day:

- Carob

- Stevia

- Blackstrap molasses

- Bone broth

- Mustard

- Flavored extracts (ex. almond, vanilla)

- Garlic

- Ginger

- Fresh or dried herbs (for example, dill, basil, chives, cilantro, mint, oregano, rosemary, sage, thyme, etc.)

- Horseradish

- Cacao (powder/nibs)

- Hot sauce

- Lemon

- Lime

- Luo han guo (monk fruit extract)

- Liquid amino acid

- Miso

- Salsa, unsweetened

- Soy sauce/tamari

- Fresh or dried spices (for example, chili powder, cardamom, cinnamon, cumin, curry, garlic powder, ginger powder, onion powder, paprika, pepper, turmeric, etc.)

- Tomato sauce, unsweetened

- Kinds of vinegar: unsweetened, organic apple cider, balsamic, red wine, white wine

- Limiting the allowed sweetner to 1–2 servings per day to reduce cravings for sweet-tasting food

Foods to Enjoy Occasionally

Legumes

Serving size:

Different kinds of beans (black-eyed, black, cannellini, edamame, garbanzo, kidney, lima, mung, navy, pinto, etc.): 1⁄2cup cooked

Beans, vegetarian refried: 1⁄2 cup

Bean soups, homemade: 3⁄4 cup

Hummus: 4 Tbsp.

Lentils (brown, green, red, yellow, French): 1⁄2 cup, cooked

Peas (pigeon, split): 1⁄2 cup, cooked

1 serving = approx. 100 calories

Macronutrients: carbohydrate = 15 g, protein = 7 g, fat = 0-3 g

Berries

Serving size:

Blackberries: 3⁄4 cup

Blueberries: 3⁄4 cup

Boysenberries: 3⁄4 cup

Cranberries, unsweetened: 1⁄2 cup

Loganberries: 3⁄4 cup

Raspberries: 1 cup

Strawberries: 11⁄4 cup

1 serving = approx. 60 calories

Macronutrients: carbohydrates = 15 g, protein = 0 g, fat = 0 g

Foods to Avoid

- Processed foods with sugar or sauces. For example, soda, fruit juice, smoothies, ice cream, candies, etc.

- Products made from wheat, grains and starches. For example, rice, pasta, cereal, etc.

- As much as possible, avoid fruits due to their high sugar content. However, you may have a limited amount of berries.

- Starchy or root vegetables should be avoided. These include tubers such as potatoes, carrots, sweet potatoes and yam.

Foods such as these have high levels of carbohydrates.

- Try not to purchase and eat foods that advertise that they are low fat of they are diet products that will help you lose weight.

- Unhealthy fats. Even though fats are important to the keto diet, you should try to avoid processed vegetable oils and stick to healthy saturated fats.

- Alcoholic beverages with high sugar content, for example, sweet wines and cocktails.

- You should avoid-sugar free diet foods for two main reasons. First, they are processed and may be high in sugar content. The keto diet states that processed food should be avoided as much as possible. Second, they are loaded with artificial sweeteners like aspartame, acesulfame K, and sucralose (such as in Diet Coke, Splenda, Sweet 'n Low).

- Pizza, Pasta, Burgers and other forms of fast food.

What Happens if I Cheat?

You are human and you may sometimes fail. However, you are able to pick yourself up after you have "fallen from the horse." Eating something that you should not in a keto diet is something that can happen to anyone. Probably this is something that everyone following the diet has done. However, the result of this "cheat" is dependent on how far along you are in the stage of ketosis or how much your body is able to convert fat into energy.

If you cheat in the early stages of the diet (after going two to three weeks without carbs), then you may have to start the process all over. Some people will never enter ketosis because they do not have the patience to do without carbs for an extended period of time (three to eight weeks). It just requires will power and the ability to stay focused as the keto diet isn't one that is difficult to adhere to. Whenever you cheat, no matter at what stage of ketosis, it will be more challenging than before. For example, eating a slice of pizza will cause you to begin to crave carbs more. Then your desire will urge you to eat anything with carbs such as cookies, buns, crackers and so on. This is just the result of this cheat and you do not really have any control over this. The urge of your body then supersedes your will power.

A duration of at least two to three weeks of no carbs is needed to get your body back into the state of ketosis that it was in. So, you should try not to focus on when you have cheated and strayed away from your diet. Be more so concerned about your healthy choices as you are eating naturally and healthily. This should put you in a good mood. One motivational idea is from a post by Kassie Ewers in a Facebook group. She stated that: "Every time I see someone eating fries or something else I can't eat, I look down and wiggle my toes and think, 'Yeah. Toes are better than fries.'" You should remember that other than weight loss, your goal is to ensure that you do not fall ill and develop ailments such as diabetes, renal failure, heart attack, stroke, hypertension, fatty liver, dementia, Alzheimer's or cancer. Those should be realistic goals and weight loss and fitness are just the natural side-effects of good health.

For support and help with staying motivated, seek out forums that discuss the keto diet. Support groups are made up of many types of people who are on different stages of their keto journey and can provide guidance and support throughout the process. You can also share your experiences and motivate others through their journey.

CHAPTER FOUR - AVOIDING OF THE KETO FLU

What is Keto Flu?

Remember we mentioned the effects of the keto flu when you have just begun the diet? While you will remember that the keto flu happens commonly to the beginners of the keto diet due to low levels of sodium and electrolytes, you may experience some flu-like symptoms including:

• Fatigue

• Headaches

• Cough

• Sniffles

• Irritability

• Nausea

Though it may feel like flu, don't be alarmed, it's not a virus and it's not contagious.

Why Does It Happen?

Since the keto diet is a diuretic, you will be losing fluids in the early stages and you will be losing electrolytes and sodium. The fact that you will be eliminating processed foods (with high sodium content) from your diet and will be eating more whole, natural foods, then your sodium intake will decrease. Also, due to the reduction of carbs, your insulin levels will also reduce the amount of sodium that's stored in your kidneys.

Ending the Keto Flu

Though it is a typical side effect of starting a keto diet, you can alleviate some if not all of the symptoms of the keto flu. The most important thing for you to do is to increase the intake of sodium and electrolytes in your body. So, how are the ways you can do this:

1, Just sprinkle some more salt on your food

2. Drink a soup broth. This normally has a high sodium content.

3. You can also eat more foods (that are acceptable for the keto diet) that are salty. Try some bacon as well as some pickled vegetables.

So, the overall advice is simply to consume more sodium at the start of the diet, and this will help to prevent the flu and all the associated symptoms. Even if you "catch" it, the symptoms are temporary and after some time they will go away and you will start your journey into the state of ketosis.

Electrolytes

Other than increasing sodium intake, you may also put back the minerals known as electrolytes into your body. During the keto diet, your kidneys will increase the rate of the process of removing the salts from your diet. Therefore, you may lose potassium and magnesium. How will you know that you have a deficiency of these nutrients? You may feel cramps in your legs, experience insomnia, nausea and other electrolyte deficiency symptoms.

We know that the brands Gatorade and Powerade are very effective drinks to help to replace electrolytes in your body, but they should be avoided because they are also laden with sugars and thus, carbs which you seek to avoid. So, how about creating your own electrolyte replacement drink (which you can name as your "keto-ade" which you can carry with you and sip on throughout the day.

You will need Morton Lite-Salt is 1/2 sodium and 1/2 potassium.

A sample recipe includes:

• 24 oz filtered water (or tap water)

• 1/4 Teaspoon Morton's Lite Salt

• 1/2 Tablespoon Magnesium Citrate (found with laxatives)

After mixing the ingredient, you should refrigerate for the best taste. Again, you should avoid sugar-free sweeteners. But if you desire to, ensure that you self-test (which will be explained soon) so as to identify your bodily reactions to these sweeteners.

Sweeteners

Here's a shortlist of artificial sweeteners you may consider using.

• Xylitol

• Erythritol

• Stevia

• Maltitol

• Sorbitol

• Sucralose (Splenda)

• Aspartame (Equal)

• Saccharine (Sweet and Low)

Note that some of these sweeteners are poisonous and can increase your risk of cancer. For example, Saccharine causes cancer. Aspartame which is found in many of our favorite diet drinks is linked to all kinds of neurological disorders. Even though they may not raise your blood sugar level, they will still affect your body's response to insulin.

The one which is most poisonous is Xylitol. It is actually poisonous to dogs and will lead to premature death. Erythritol/Stevia combination like Swerve is one type that many people like and Sorbitol has a cooling effect that may not be liked by everybody. As stated before, do self-testing as it reported by some that Maltitol lowers their levels of ketosis and may cause diarrhea.

Self-Testing

Even though there are restrictions on this diet, there are fundamental foods that are acceptable which do not raise the insulin level in your blood, especially not to the point where it is detrimental to your health. These foods include fats and proteins (but you still need to be cognizant not to exceed the daily amount). These also include minerals, pure vitamins and green leafy vegetables. Our bodies are different so surely, certain types of food that affect us will differ For example, dairy, artificial sweeteners, nuts, alcohol can affect our bodies differently. Therefore, for you to truly follow the keto diet, you need to be able to test yourself. You can do so by using a Blood Glucose Meter.

If you are unable to afford or readily access a blood glucose meter, you may need to test your food manually (by yourself. This is a time-consuming process. One such indicator to track how you react to foods is the craving you have or the weight you have gained when you weigh the next day after consuming the food. Even though this is not entirely accurate, you can use it to test if you should consume the food again based on the effect it has on your sugar levels.

Testing is very important especially when you have reached a plateau which can make you very frustrated as you can't understand why your weight is not going down any further. So, finding out the foods that affect you or makes your blood sugar or insulin level to rise will make a difference in your weight loss plan. Therefore, check to see what foods are good for you to eat and omit those from your diet as they may negatively affect your weight loss plan.

Glucose Curve

A glucose curve can be performed on any food type. There are two questions that you need to answer in this process:

How quickly will the food I have eaten convert into glucose in my blood?

Will my body release insulin to deal with the glucose from the foods eaten?

After you have eaten something that has spiked your insulin level and thus, your blood sugar level, your levels will normally return to the norm after 2 – 3 hours. Those with Type 2 diabetes may take up to 5 hours for their blood sugar level to go back to being normal. Exercise may also affect this. So, give your body some time (at least an hour) after light exercise or maybe several hours if you have had an extreme workout. Upon waking in the mornings, your body uses hormones to help boost your production of glucose. So, the best time to perform this check is a few hours after waking up and you have skipped breakfast.

What To Expect

You are by now eager to start the keto diet – be on your way to successfully lose weight. However, it is suggested that before you begin, it is best that you visit your general practitioner or even a nutritionist. In this visit, you will need to inform him/her about your desire to start on the keto diet plan and complete a blood profile. This profile will include data related to your insulin levels, liver function, and vitamins and nutrients that your body may be lacking.

Your doctor may not agree with the diet due to ideas that are related to the negative views they have about fat and cholesterol. You will just need to use scientific evidence to support your argument. If the doctor continues to persist and state that you should not cut carbs out of your diet, then you may need to choose another doctor.

Since we know that weight loss is not only about the number on the scale and will also include the circumference of your body, you will not weigh yourself as well as take measurements. Most importantly, measure the circumference of your waist. The decrease in circumference is a very good indicator that you are seeing results.

Also, consider stocking up on Omega-3 supplements as well as multivitamins. The test that was mentioned before will determine if you need a vitamin D supplement. This is necessary as research as shown that a lot of people lack this nutrient in their bodies. It is during week one of two strict adherence to the meal plan that you may experience keto flu as previously discussed in the chapter. You may go ahead and reread about these symptoms that you may experience as well as the ways of alleviating them.

However, you may get a rash when beginning the keto diet. This is normally known as a keto rash. Why does this occur? Because of the candida or yeast in your skin dying off due to the change in diet. This is a harmless process and the yeast reacts this way to ketones and such it may leave your skin feeling itchy. This as well does not last very long and simple topical creams such as calamine lotion or hydrocortisone can be applied to the skin to treat the symptoms.

After these symptoms dissipate, you are on your way to experiencing steady weight loss. But beware – eventually you will hit a plateau. This means that you will stop experiencing weight loss as before.

This can happen for numerous reasons. How do you react to this? The initial response is to do nothing. Just focus on the idea that your body is still burning fat, your blood sugar levels are declining the triglycerides as well in your blood. Also consider the fact that your blood pressure has decreased and it is maintained at the optimal level.

So, note that your lean muscle mass is increasing and so stop worrying about the fact that you have plateaued. Consider your measurements are steadily decreasing. Noe the muscle I denser than fat and so a small mass of muscle weighs more than fat of the same weight. Therefore, as you are losing weight, you will also be gaining muscles, so your weight loss may stop or even slow. Just don't worry and enjoy the numerous other benefits that you can achieve from your keto diet.

However, you can combat this plateau. If you experience it within the third of eight weeks of adhering to the keto diet, then you may need to consider fasting. Try eating only one meal per day without no snacking but however drinking water and also fluids to replace the electrolytes lost. Have coffee with no sweeteners or cream. After some time, you will recognize that you do not feel hungry and you actually feel great. You may be wondering which meals will be omitted and which mealtime will remain, This is dependent on you. Some people will only eat a late lunch and others may eat dinner. Again, the choice is yours; choose what suits you and your lifestyle best.

CHAPTER FIVE – KETOGENIC MEAL PLANS AND RECIPES

In planning a meal plan that adheres to the rules of the keto diet, one needs to ensure that there are many servings of oils and fats, nuts and seeds and varied sources of protein. Also include the recommended servings of vegetables – remember to choose the non-starchy varieties. These vegetables will be your keep source of fiber, phytonutrients and the necessary vitamins and minerals that are needed for maintaining a healthy body.

Meal Plan for the Fast Food Junkie

Maybe you have a very busy schedule and you are unable to put the effort into creating a meal that adheres to the keto diet. You may even have the financial resources to be able to eat out. If you are desirous to see immediate results, there is actually a no-fail one-week plan that is well suited for you.

For such a plan you will need to purchase:

- Some brand of low carb bread (Mahler is a good brand to use)

- Cheese crisps (made with cheese only)

- Ketchup which has no sugar added

- Apple cider vinegar

- A bottle of coconut oil

For best storage to allow the bread to last longer, keep it in the freezer. Also, you can travel with your cheese crisps anywhere and snack on them.

Breakfast

In the mornings, you will need to toast the slices of Mahler's bread and butter them. You may wrap them and then you are on your way through the door. You may then go through the McDonald's drive-thru and purchase two breakfast bagels you like with extra cheese. These bagels will come with bacon, egg and cheese; sausage, egg, and cheese; or steak, egg and cheese). You can mix it up by making different choices each day. You will not be eating the bagel itself, so replace the bagel with your toast. Therefore, you will be putting the proteins between your own slices of toasted bread. You may also get yourself a coffee or tea. Heavy cream is okay, but do not add any sugar. Yes, sugar substitutes may be used, it is recommended that you avoid them as much as possible (refer to the list of things to avoid in a previous chapter). Also, avoid milk. You can replace it with half and half. Other foods to avoid are pancakes and other food items that contain starches and sugars. Those two bagels will be enough to keep you full until the next meal.

Lunch

When it is lunchtime, you should have your two slices of low-carb bread on hand. You can toast it the same and add mayo and ketchup too it. Remember that the ketchup should be one in which no sugar is added. You then go to your favorite burger joint and order two burgers. It's okay to request some extra mayonnaise, cheese, lettuce, pickles, mustard, tomatoes or even mushroom. Don't forget that extra bacon is good too. If the restaurant has or if you have carries your own sugar-free ketchup, load up on that as well. Remember when ordering, tell them to hold the ketchup and onions. It is better that you sprinkle the bread with onion powder if this is something that you like the taste of. Just remember to avoid fries, soda or anything with sugar, but extra bacon and cheese, please!

With all you have consumed, you must be thirsty. This means that you will have water on hand. Even though you can purchase a bottle anywhere you go, you can also have a water bottle in which you add a teaspoon of apple cider vinegar. This concoction will be refreshing and is also known to lower insulin levels.

Dinner

You have been doing great so far and it's now time for dinner. Why not treat yourself to a meal at one of your favorite restaurants. Ensure that you finish the meal before 7PM and eat nothing else for the rest of the night. It will be great to order a salad as this is on the menu of most restaurants. Just avoid the croutons (this is bread and thus, added carbohydrates). When choosing salad dressing, choose ones that are not "sweet" and have much-added sugars (no thousand island and French salad dressings). Blue cheese dressing is a good option.

Order some wine as well. If choosing a red wine, pinot noir is a great option. If you prefer white wine, you can choose a good brand of pinot grigio. Probably you are a fan of hard liquor such as rum, vodka or bourbon. It is okay to order those as well. However, do not overdo it. Limit yourself to one and use chasers that do not have sugars.

There are quite a few dinner options you can choose from when eating out while still adhering to the principles of the keto diet. These include:

Buffalo Wings. Restaurants such as Chili's has options such as "wings over buffalo" or "smoked wings" which do not use a sauce in their preparation.

You can definitely order a steak. However, when ordering, ask for the fattier cuts: prime rib, ribeye, etc. it's best to avoid the leaner cuts of meat such as filet mignon. Ensure to ask for extra butter to melt over it. Order a big one if you are extra hungry. Tell the waiter to hold the potatoes. You may replace the potatoes with vegetables. Broccoli and spinach are good options.

Salmon. Ask that your salmon filet or steak is cooked in a lot of butter or oil.

Shrimp Scampi. Again, ask that your shrimp are swimming in butter and garlic. You can even have two servings but avoid having the pasta.

Pork Chops, Lamb Shank, Beef Short Ribs are also good choices. As always, avoid the carbs; so, you will not be consuming any of their free breadsticks nor any of the mashed potatoes. Most restaurants are accommodating so you may ask them not to cut the fat from your meat when preparing your meal. You should also remember to eat all of the fat off your meat. Don't cut it away.

The Next Morning

You can follow the plans for the morning as stated previously. But here is some additional guidelines which may be useful to you. When having your coffee, you may place four cups in your blender with a heaping spoon of coconut oil and flavor it with some cinnamon, nutmeg, vanilla, or any other flavoring you want. You can blend everything together and then enjoy. The coconut oil will leave you feeling satiated and you should be able to go a long time without getting hungry. If you are not hungry at lunchtime; skip it. This will not negatively affect your diet. Remember it was stated that fasting on this diet is also beneficial. The aim is to follow what your body is telling you. So, if you are hungry eat, but ensure that you stop when you are full. The use of coconut oil in your coffee can help you with those cravings. So, maybe it will be good to have that in the morning and afternoons, before a meal. Carbs are very addictive. If you rid yourself of carbs, you are better able to read the signals that your body sends – to tell you when you are full or hungry. Over time, when you follow those signals, you will be able to have control over what you eat and how much.

Sample Diet Plans

So, you have been considering meals you can consume when following the keto diet. Probably you would like some recipes that you can follow. Preparing a meal plan on a keto diet may vary. One such way in which people plan a keto diet is to consider a light breakfast with lunch and dinner. Below we will discuss a 3 Day Ketogenic Diet Plan.

Planning for meals within the parameter of the keto diet may seem hard but we have made this easy for you. You will be provided with meals and simple recipes that you can follow in this chapter.

Getting Started

To get started on your journey of eating healthily by following the keto diet, you need to simply remove those foods that do not adhere to the plan. So, best is that you clear your kitchen of those "forbidden" food items and buying those that are good for your weight loss plan. You may donate unwanted foodstuff to charity instead of letting them go to waste.

3 Day Meal Plan

In the 3 Day Meal Plan, you will be provided with meal ideas for breakfast, lunch, dinner and then a light snack.

Day 1

<u>Breakfast</u>

Scrambled Egg and Yogurt

Ingredients

- 1 whole egg

- 1 1/2 tsp. almond butter

- 1 tsp. extra virgin olive oil

- 6 almonds

- 1/2 cup plain Greek yogurt

[Calories: 336, Fat: 25 g, Carbohydrate: 9 g, Protein 21 g]

Directions: pour olive oil in a pan and then scramble the egg. Add Greek yogurt and almond butter, and crushed almonds on the side.

Lunch

Chia Keto and Spinach Shake

Ingredient

- 3 Tbsp. light canned coconut milk

- 2 scoops keto shake powder

- 1 Tbsp. chia seeds

- 2 cups spinach

[Calories: 354, Fat: 24 g, Carbohydrate: 14 g, Protein 25 g]

Directions: blend ingredients with water and ice until you achieve the desired consistency.

Dinner

Tuna Wrap

Ingredients

- 2 oz. canned tuna (in oil or water)

- 1/2 cup shredded green pepper

- 2 Tbsp. unsweetened avocado mayonnaise

- 1 cup romaine lettuce (2 large leaves)

- 1 Tbsp. pine nuts

[Calories: 328, Fat: 31 g, Carbohydrate: 6 g, Protein 13 g]

Directions: place all ingredients (except lettuce, in a bowl and mix them. Wrap the mixture in lettuce leaves.

Snacks

Nut Butter and Celery

Ingredients

- 3 tsp. almond butter

- 1 cup celery, cut into strips

[Calories: 114, Fat: 9 g, Carbohydrate: 6 g, Protein 4 g]

Directions: spread the nut butter on celery or dip the celery in the nut butter.

Keto Almond Shake

Ingredients

- Water (depends on the consistency and taste you desire)

- Ice

- 2 scoops keto shake powder

- 3 tsp. almond butter

- 6 almonds

- 1 Tbsp. MCT powder

[Calories: 460, Fat: 36 g, Carbohydrate: 12 g, Protein 26 g]

Directions: blend all ingredients with ice and water until the desired consistency is reached.

Day 2

Breakfast

Keto Coffee Shake

Ingredients

- Water (depends on the consistency and taste you desire)

- Ice

- 2 scoops keto shake powder

- 1½ Tbsp. ground flaxseeds

- 1 tsp. heavy cream

- 4 oz. coffee

[Calories: 302, Fat: 21 g, Carbohydrate: 8 g, Protein 22 g]

Directions: blend all ingredients with ice and water until the desired consistency is reached.

<u>Lunch</u>

Salmon Salad

Ingredients

- 1/2 tomato

- 1/4 cucumber

- 1 cup kale

- 1 cup spinach

- 1/4 onion

- 4 Tbsp. avocado

- 1½ oz. smoked salmon

[Calories: 220, Fat: 9 g, Carbohydrate: 19 g, Protein 20 g]

Directions: prep all ingredients (cut or chop) and place all ingredients in a bowl and mix them. Then add salt and pepper as desired squeeze in some lime juice.

Dinner

Chicken Salad

Ingredients

- 1/2 oz. chicken, shredded

- 6 walnut halves

- 2 tbsp. unsweetened avocado mayonnaise

- 1/2 cup celery, chopped

- 1/2 cup cucumber, chopped

Directions: place all ingredients in a bowl, mix and serve.

[Calories: 399, Fat: 36 g, Carbohydrate: 6 g, Protein 20 g]

Snacks

Creamy Avocado Dip with Cucumbers

Ingredients

- 1 cup cucumbers (peel and slice into strips)

- 4 Tbsp. avocado

- 1 Tbsp. cream cheese

Directions: mash the avocado in a bowl and then mix in the cream cheese. You may spread the mixture on the cucumber. You may also use the mash as a dip.

[Calories: 118, Fat: 10 g, Carbohydrate: 6 g, Protein 2 g]

Keto Coconut Shake

Ingredients

- Water (depends on the consistency and taste you desire)

- Ice

- 2 scoops keto shake powder

- 1½ Tbsp. unsweetened, shredded coconut

- 3 Tbsp. light canned coconut milk

Directions: blend all ingredients with ice and water until the desired consistency is reached.

[Calories: 311, Fat: 22g, Carbohydrate: 11 g, Protein 21 g]

Day 3

Breakfast

Egg Salad

Ingredients

- 1 boiled whole egg (cut into bite-sized pieces)

- A sprinkle of chopped green onion

- 2 Tbsp. avocado

[Calories: 308, Fat: 31 g, Carbohydrate: 0 g, Protein 9 g]

Directions: mix all the ingredients together in a bowl. You may serve it on some lettuce.

Lunch

Chicken Salad

Ingredients

- 1/2 oz. chicken, shredded

- 1/2 cup celery, chopped

- 6 walnut halves

- 1⁄2 cup cucumber, chopped

- 2 tbsp. unsweetened avocado mayonnaise

Directions: place ingredients in a bowl and mix them, then serve.

[Calories: 399, Fat: 36 g, Carbohydrate: 6 g, Protein 20 g]

Dinner

Keto Chia Shake

Ingredients

- Water (depends on the consistency and taste you desire)

- Ice

- 2 scoops keto shake powder

- 2 Tbsp. chia seeds

Directions: Blend all ingredients with ice and water until the desired consistency is reached.

[Calories: 358, Fat: 23 g, Carbohydrate: 17 g, Protein 25 g]

Snacks

Crunchy Vegetables

Ingredients

- 2 Tbsp. avocado

- 3⁄4 cup celery, cut into strips

- 1⁄4 cup cucumbers, diced

Directions: In a bowl, mash the avocado and mix in cucumbers. You may spread the mixture on the celery or use the mixture as a dip.

[Calories: 80, Fat: 6 g, Carbohydrate: 6 g, Protein 2 g]

Keto Pumpkin Shake

Ingredients

- Water (depends on the consistency and taste you desire)

- Ice

- 2 scoops keto shake powder

- 2 tsp. cream

- 1 Tbsp. pumpkin seeds

- 1 tsp. pumpkin pie spice

Directions: Blend all ingredients with ice and water until the desired consistency is reached.

[Calories: 317, Fat: 22 g, Carbohydrate: 9 g, Protein 25 g]

Additional Ideas Suitable for Ketogenic Meal Plan

Here are some additional meals that you can eat while following a keto diet:

- Prawn avocado salad

- Keto shake (made with coconut milk and MCT oil)

- Raw vegetable Pad Thai

- Curried tofu

- Mediterranean salad

- Herbed baked salmon

- Seasoned chicken with shredded cabbage

- Thai lime and sesame stir-fry

- Eggs Florentine

- Keto coffee

- Keto shake using MCT oil and coconut milk

- Zesty Mexican keto soup

- Cheesy scrambled eggs

- Mini frittatas with spinach and tomato

Though snacking is not encouraged. You may snack on healthy food options. These should include protein, fat and carbohydrate-based on the macronutrients consumed in the other meals. Examples of snacks are:

- 1-2 celery stalks with 1 Tbsp. nut butter

- 4 oz. Greek yogurt with 3⁄4 cup blueberries

- 1 cup of either sliced peppers, cauliflower (raw), celery, or broccoli

- 2 Tbsp. hummus

- 1⁄2 medium tomato with 2 Tbsp. avocado

- 1 Tbsp. toasted pumpkin seeds (pepitas) with 1⁄2 cup cottage cheese

Breakfast Recipes

Although we have highlighted some meal ideas in the 3 Deal Meal Plan. Here are some other breakfast recipes that you could try.

Avocado Bun Breakfast Burger

Macronutrients per serving: 717 calories, 61.36g fat, 20.11g carbs, 14.6g fiber, 2.88g sugar, 27.41g protein

Ingredients

- 1 avocado

- 1 egg

- 1 tbsp olive oil

- 1 breakfast sausage

- 1 lettuce leaf

- 1 slice tomato

- 1 tbsp mayo

- pinch of salt and pepper

- sesame seeds

Directions: cut avocado uniformly. Preheat oil in a non-stick skillet. Ensure that it is at roughly medium heat. Cook sausage for at least one minute on each side then remove from the pan. Lower the heat and then crack an egg in the pot. Cook to your desired style. In serving, place avocado on the plate and then some mayo. Top everything with lettuce, tomato, sausage and place the egg on the top. If desired sprinkle some salt, pepper and sesame seeds.

Breakfast Sausage, Eggs and Greens

Macronutrients per serving: 560 calories – 43.30g fat, 12g carbs, 7g fiber, 2.79g sugar, 31.71g protein

Ingredients

- 1 breakfast sausage

- 2 eggs

- 4 broccoli florets (50g)

- green beans

- 1.5 tbsp olive oil

- 1 garlic clove

- pinch salt and pepper,

- garlic powder

Directions: prep the green beans by removing the stems. Then mince the garlic. Bring some water to boil in a pot. Boil the broccoli and green beans and cook until the vegetable are tender. Once cooked, remove from the pot and place them on a plate. Add olive oil to a hot frying pan. Place the breakfast sausage in the pan and allow it to toast on both sides. After they are thoroughly cooked, remove them from the pan and add the eggs. Scramble eggs and then place them on the plate with the sausage. Using the same frying pan, add green beans and garlic and fry until crisp. Sprinkle salt and pepper to your desired taste preference and then serve.

90-sec Sausage Egg McMuffin

Macronutrients per serving: 719 calories – 60.15g fat, 9.38g carbs, 4.15g fiber, 2.61g sugar, 36.57g protein

Ingredients

- 1 breakfast sausage

- 1 slice tomato

- 1 egg

- 1 tsp olive oil

- 1 tsp mayo

90-sec bread:

- 1 tbsp refined coconut oil

- 1 egg

- 1/2 tsp salt

- 1/2 tsp baking powder

- 3 tbsp almond flour

Directions: place the ingredients for the 90-second bread into a large mug, mix thoroughly and then microwave for 90 seconds. Let the mug cool before trying to remove it. After this, you should carefully slice it in two. Heat a frying pan and then add olive oil. When the oil is hot, place in breakfast sausage and cook each side thoroughly. Place the slices of the bread on a grill until both sides are toasted to your desire. Cook the eggs based on your desired style. Place mayonnaise on the bread, then the tomato slice, egg and then cover with the last slice of bread.

Spinach and Pork Omelet

Macronutrients per serving: 446 calories – 34.96g fat 4.29g carbs 0.9g fiber, 3.39g sugar, 27.84g protein

Ingredients (2 portions)

- 1 breakfast sausage

- 6 eggs

- 1 cup fresh spinach (30g)

- 1/4 red pepper (40g)

- 2 garlic cloves

- 2 tbsp olive oil

- 1/4 tsp salt and pepper

- garlic powder

- parsley

Directions: break up the sausage into a crumble. Mince the garlic and slice the red peppers into bite-size pieces. Heat a non-stick frying pan. Add the olive oil and wait until its heated. While cooking the sausage add the minced garlic, chopped red pepper and spinach. Allow the spinach to cook until soft. This may take one to two minutes. Crack the eggs in a large bowl and add spices to your desired taste. Whisk ingredients for two minutes. Pour out all the egg mixture into the pan and let it cook for 4-5 minutes. When the top of the omelet is cooked through, slide it into a plate and cut in half. You may save the other half for another meal.

Avocado Boat, Sausage and Asparagus

Macronutrients per serving: 537 calories − 42.29g, fat 11.2g, carbs 8.3g fiber, 1.3g sugar, 30.78g protein

Ingredients

60g sausage

1-2 asparagus

1 tsp olive oil

1/2 avocado

70g tuna

1/4 cup wilted spinach (50g fresh)

1 tbsp mayo

pinch salt and pepper

Directions: heat frying pan and then add olive oil. You should fry sausages and asparagus until they are cooked well. Serve them on a plate. Slice and cut avocado into cubes and place in the bowl with the tuna, wilted spinach, mayo and desired salt and pepper. Serve in the avocado skin/shell and place it on the plate with the sausages and asparagus.

Eggs, Bacon and Tomato Salad

Macronutrients per serving: 541 calories – 39.81g fat, 8.12g carbs, 1.8g fiber, 4.42g sugar, 36.3g protein

Ingredients

3 slices bacon

2 eggs

1/4 red pepper

1/4 zucchini (40g)

pinch salt and pepper

3 slices tomato

1 basil leaf

1 tsp olive oil

1 garlic clove

1/2 tsp vinegar

Directions: slice the red pepper and zucchini and then fry the bacon until crispy. Remove the bacon from the pot and place it on a plate. Place the peppers and zucchini in the frying pan with the bacon fat and cook until they are tender. Crack the eggs open and scramble with the pepper and zucchini until cooked. Sprinkle the salt and pepper to your taste. Put on the plate with the bacon. After mincing the garlic clove and basil leaf, mix in a small bowl along with the olive oil, basil, garlic, vinegar, salt and pepper. Place the tomato into the mix and ensure that they are coated with the mixture.

Avocado Boat, Sausages and Scrambled Eggs

Macronutrients per serving: 792 calories – 64.82g fat, 11.23g carbs, 7.5g fiber

Ingredients

60g sausage

2 eggs

2 mushrooms

1/4 spinach

1 tbsp olive oil

pinch salt and pepper

1/2 avocado

70g tuna can

1 tbsp mayo

1 tsp sliced green onion

Direction: slice the mushrooms. Fry the sausages in oil until thoroughly cooked, add them to a plate. Fry the mushrooms and fresh spinach until soft and add the eggs to that mixed. Scramble your eggs, adding salt and black pepper to your taste. Place scrambled eggs on a plate.

After removing the avocado from the skin, mash it and mix with mayo, salt and pepper, tuna and green peppers in a bowl. Place mixture in the skin of the avocado and then place it on the plate.

Lunch Recipes

Avocado Cream and Zoodles

Macronutrients per serving: 383 calories – 35.34g fat, 18g carbs, 9.4g fiber, 5.46g protein

Ingredients

1 zucchini

1/2 avocado (100g)

20 basil leaves

1.5 tbsp olive oil

3 brown mushrooms (30g)

1 garlic clove

1 tsp lemon juice

1/4 tsp salt

Directions: Spiralize your zucchini and slice the mushrooms in half. Add the avocado, basil, 1 tbsp olive oil, garlic, lemon juice and salt in a cup. Blend with a stick blender for about a minute until everything is super creamy and delicious. Heat frying pan and then add olive oil. Cook mushrooms in the oil until they are tender. Place zucchini noodle into the pan and only cook until it is heated. Add the avocado cream and mix well, then serve.

BLT Lettuce Boats

Macronutrients per serving: 362 calories – 33.20g fat, 10.64g carbs, 3.34g fiber, 1.79g sugar, 8.62g protein

Ingredients

2 lettuce leaves

2 slices bacon

1/2 avocado

1/4 tomato

1 tbsp mayo

Directions: Fry the bacon until crispy. Slice the tomato into a few slices. Slice the avocado. Spread mayonnaise on each leaf of lettuce, then add the avocado, tomato and bacon.

Rosemary Chicken and Broccoli

Macronutrients per serving: 461 calories – 33.71g fat, 6.99g carbs, 2.8g fiber, 1.7g sugar, 33.94g protein

Ingredients

1 boneless chicken leg (125g)

1/3 broccoli head (100g)

1/4 tsp salt

1/4 tsp black pepper

1/2 tsp rosemary

1 tbsp olive oil

2 tbsp water

Direction: Clean chicken and then cut in small pieces. Season with salt and pepper. Pick apart broccoli into florets. Heat olive oil in a cast-iron skillet. Place in the chicken along with the rosemary. Fry chicken until fully cooked and crisp on all sides (about three minutes). Place broccoli florets into the pot and cook for about a minute. Ensure to mix everything together. Add water and let the broccoli steam until tender.

Zucchini Salad w/ Grilled Chicken Thigh

Macronutrients per serving: 430 calories – 36.93g fat, 8.18g carbs, 2.6g fiber, 2.82g sugar, 22.64g protein

Ingredients

1/4 zucchini

1/4 red pepper

50g swiss chard

1/4 tomato

5 basil leaves

1 tbsp olive oil

1 tsp vinegar

1 garlic clove

1/4 tsp salt and pepper

1 chicken thigh with skin (75g)

1 tbsp olive oil

1/2 tsp salt and pepper

Directions: Use a peeler to make long ribbons of zucchini. Prepare the other vegetables: chop the peppers and the swish chard; dice the tomatoes; mince garlic cloves and basil leaves. Mix all the vegetables together with vinegar, olive oil, salt and pepper in a bowl.

Then serve on a plate. Season the chicken thigh using the salt and pepper. Preheat a skillet and add oil. Place in the chicken thigh with the skin side down first. Cook until crispy and then flip to cook the other side. Cook until the chicken is tender and cooked through. Serve it on the plate with the salad.

Rosemary Shrimps and Radishes

Macronutrients per serving: 261 calories – 15.63g fat, 8.13g carbs, 3.2g fiber, 3.89g sugar, 17.84g protein

Ingredients

5 radishes (85g)

10 shrimps (100g)

3 broccoli florets (60g)

1 tbsp rosemary

1 tbsp olive oil

1/2 tsp salt, pepper

Directions: Place broccoli into boiling water. Cook until tender. Heat a frying pan and then add the olive oil. Place both shrimp and radishes in the pan. Ensure to place them separately. Add salt and pepper to your desired taste. Then add some rosemary. Cook everything for a few minutes until the radishes are soft and the shrimps become pink in color.

Chicken Brochettes and Easy Salad

Macronutrients per serving: 400 calories − 26.29g fat, 13.28g carbs, 4.2g fiber, 5.89g sugar, 27.92g protein

Ingredients

3 chicken brochettes

5 lettuce leaves

1/4 red pepper

1 slice tomato

1 tbsp sesame dressing

Directions: rip the lettuce into bite-size pieces. Slice the red pepper and tomato. Add the sesame dressing and coat well. Serve the salad and add the chicken brochettes on top.

Kale Beef and Veggie Caesar Wrap

Macronutrients per serving: 714 calories − 59.64g fat, 17.23g carbs, 8.6g fiber, 2.66g sugar, 30.93g protein

Ingredients

1 portion Caesar dressing

1 large kale leaf (50g)

1/2 avocado

1/2 tomato

1/8 red onion

100g thinly sliced beef

1 tbsp olive oil

1/4 tsp salt, pepper, garlic powder

Direction: carefully trim the stem of the kale leaf so that you can roll the leaf to make a sandwich. Slice the avocado, red onion and tomato. Heat a skillet and then add olive oil. Place in the beef and season with salt pepper, and garlic powder. Cook beef until tender and cook thoroughly. This may take one to two minutes. Spread the Caesar dressing on the kale leaf and then add toppings to one side. Carefully roll the leaf until you have made a wrap. To prevent the wrap from unraveling, place in aluminum foil or place toothpicks to secure the end.

Dinner Recipes

Chicken Cutlet and Cauli Rice

Macronutrients per serving: 665 calories – 42.35g fat, 14.64g carbs, 8g fiber, 4.54g sugar, 58.04g protein

Ingredients (2 portions)

1 small cauliflower (300g)

2 tbsp sesame oil

1 tbsp coconut aminos

1 tsp dashi powder

1/4 tsp salt and pepper

1 skinless chicken breast (260g)

pinch salt and pepper

1 egg

4 tbsp almond flour

40g pork rinds

pinch salt and pepper

oil (coconut oil is best)

Direction: use the food processor to rice the cauliflower. If you do not have a food processor, you may use a cheese grater. Heat sesame oil in a wok and place in the riced cauliflower. Cook the cauliflower for a few minutes; after that, add dashi, salt and pepper and the coconut aminos. Mix everything together until thoroughly combined. Continue frying until the cauliflower is cooked and a bit crunchy. Crush the pork rinds by either placing it into a food processor (you may also do this with your hands. Incorporate the pork rinds into the almond flour, adding salt and pepper to taste. Then whisk an egg into a bowl.

Slice the chicken breast into strips. Season the strips using the salt and pepper and then dip them into the whisked egg. Coat the strips of chicken with the breading on both sides. Fry them in 150C/300F preheated oil until cooked thoroughly. Serve with the cauli rice. Keep half for another meal.

Roasted Chicken Leg & Veggies

Macronutrients per serving: 632 calories — 37.78g fat, 9.06g carbs, 3g fiber, 4.69g sugar, 61.15g protein

Ingredients (2 portions)

6 asparagus spears (40g) 1/2 zucchini

100g mini carrots

2 chicken legs (600g)

1 tbsp olive oil

6 cherry tomatoes (80g)

1/4 tsp salt, black pepper, cumin, paprika, chili powder

Directions: Light oven and preheat to 200C/400F. Prepare the asparagus by cutting off the stems and also slice the zucchini into strips. Cut the mini carrots in halves. Place all vegetables into a cast-iron skillet and place the chicken seasoned with salt, black pepper, cumin, paprika and chili powder on top. Bake everything in the oven for about 50 minutes uncovered. Since this is two serving. Serve half of the meal and store the other half for the next day.

Grilled Cod and Shrimps

Macronutrients per serving: 338 calories – 9.23g fat, 5.54g carbs, 1g fiber, 1.97g sugar, 55.42g protein

Ingredients (2 portions)

2 cod fillet (300g)

200g shrimps

1 tbsp lemon juice

2 stems fresh parsley

2 tbsp olive oil

2 garlic cloves

8 cherry tomatoes

Direction: mince the garlic and parsley. Heat a pan and add butter to melt. Add garlic into the melted butter and cook for a few minutes. Place the shrimp and cod into the pan and cook each for two minutes on each side. The shrimp will look pink when cooked. Try not to overcook the. Also, in flipping the cod, it may break apart, so handle gently. Add tomatoes to the pan and cook until tender. You may squeeze lemon juice over everything and then serve. Since this is two servings, you may eat half and store the other half for another meal.

Arugula Caesar Salad and Veggies

Macronutrients per serving: 259 calories – 19.62g fat, 19.08g carbs, 9.1g fiber, 7.34g sugar, 7.07g protein

Ingredients

3 leaves iceberg lettuce (120g)

40g arugula

2 asparagus (60g)

4 broccoli florets (60g)

5-6 slices cucumber (20g)

1/2 avocado

1/2 tomato

1 portion Caesar dressing

Directions: Bring water in a pot to boil and then place in broccoli. Cook broccoli until tender. Remove and then place in a bowl to cool. In another bowl place shredded arugula and lettuce. Also, add in sliced avocado, tomato and cucumber. Squeeze in salad dressing and stir until the dressing coats all the items.

Rosemary Pork Roast

Macronutrients per serving: 359 calories – 23.88g fat, 0.12g carbs, 0.1g fiber, 0g sugar, 33.75g protein

Ingredients (3 portions)

500g boneless pork roast

1 tbsp olive oil

1 tsp salt

1 tsp black pepper

1 tbsp rosemary

Directions: preheat the oven to 200C/400F. Massage the pork roast with olive oil, salt, black pepper and rosemary. Place it on a baking tray on some parchment paper. Cook in the oven for one hour. After done, cool for 5-10 minutes. Slice and serve. Keep 2/3 for the other meals.

Side Caesar Salad

Macronutrients per serving: 214 calories – 16.72g fat, 7.85g carbs, 2.6g fiber, 3.66g sugar, 8.96g protein

Ingredients

4 lettuce leaves

1 egg

1/2 tomato

3 broccoli stems (50g)

1 tbsp Caesar dressing

Direction: boil eggs for 7 minutes exactly. You are going to "shock" them to stop the cooking process. This is done by transferring them into an ice bath. After cooled, remove from the shell. Cook broccoli in boiling water until tender. Cut broccoli and eggs into bite-sized pieces and place in a bowl. Rip lettuce into small pieces and add to the picture. After adding Caesar salad dressing, mix everything well. This will be best served with a rosemary pork roast.

Bacon, Broccoli and Mushrooms

Macronutrients per serving: 386 calories – 26.22g fat, 4g carbs, 1.6g fiber, 0.98g sugar, 32.72g protein

Ingredients

- 80g broccoli

- 4 brown mushrooms (40g)

- 3 slices bacon (40g cooked)

- 1/4 tsp salt

- 1/2 tsp rosemary

- 1/4 tsp garlic powder

- pinch black pepper

Direction: bring water to boil in a small pot and place in broccoli. Cook the broccoli until tender. Sprinkle salt over the bacon slices and cut into 1cm strips and also chop mushrooms into smaller pieces. Place bacon in the pan and fry until crisp. After this, add the mushroom and cook until soft. Sprinkle in rosemary and cook for about a minute. Add the broccoli, mix everything together and sprinkle the garlic powder and black pepper over.

Dessert Recipes

<u>Cannoli Mini Cheese balls</u>

Prep Time: 10 minutes

Cook Time: 30 minutes

Servings: 8

Ingredients

- 8 ounces cream cheese softened (or mascarpone cheese)

- 1/2 cup ricotta cheese

- 1/2 cup Confectioners Swerve or equivalent

- 1 teaspoon cinnamon

   WHITE CHOCOLATE:

- 2 ounces cocoa butter

- 1/3 cup Confectioners Swerve

- 1 teaspoon vanilla extract **OR** other extracts like **MINT**

- 1/8 teaspoon sea salt

MILK CHOCOLATE BAR (ADD):

- 1/4 ounces of unsweetened baking chocolate

DARK CHOCOLATE BAR (ADD):

- 1/2 ounces of unsweetened baking chocolate 1/2 to 1 ounce, depending on how dark you like it

Directions: in a bowl mix until well combined the cream cheese, ricotta, natural sweetener and cinnamon. Scoop out only a small amount of the mixture with your hands and form it into 2-inch balls, placing each of them on a parchment-lined baking sheet. Cover the baking sheet and place in the refrigerator for at least 30 minutes.

While the balls are in the refrigerator make the coating. Using a double boiler with the heat on medium-high, fully melt the cocoa butter, then stir in natural sweetener, extracts and salt. Place the liquid into a candy bar-shaped mold (or into a

Tupperware lined with parchment paper) and cool in the refrigerator until chocolate is solid, about an hour. If you wish for the candy to form faster, you can place the molds in a freezer till they are set. When solid enough, remove from the fridge and chop into small pieces. Placing them in a bowl, roll the chilled cream cheese balls in the chocolate pieces.

Nutritional Info (per serving)

- Calories 196

- Fat 19g – 88%

- Protein 3g – 8%

- Carbs 2g – 4%

- Fiber 1g

Chocolate Puff Muffins with Custard

Prep Time: 5 minutes

Cook Time: 30 minutes

Servings: 6

Ingredients

Muffins:

- 12 egg whites

- 2 tsp cream of tartar

- 1 pinch sea salt

- 1/2 cup Jay Robb chocolate egg white protein powder

- 1 cup Confectioners Swerve

- 1/4 cup unsweetened cocoa powder

- 1 tsp chocolate extract or other extracts

Custard:

- 6 large egg yolks

- 1/4 cup coconut oil

- 1/2 cup unsweetened almond milk

- 1/4 cup Swerve

Directions: preheat your oven to 175 degrees C or 350 degrees F. Sift protein powder, cocoa powder and natural sweetener together and set aside. Crack eggs and place egg whites in a bowl. Whip them until they are light and foamy. Using a mixture will provide better results faster. The yolks will be used to make the custard so don't throw them away. Add cream of tartar into the egg whites and continue to beat until very stiff. Flavor to your desire adding your favorite extract. Then fold in the protein powder mixture quickly. Pour into greased cupcake liners. In an oven preheated at 325 degrees F (175 degrees C), bake for 30 minutes. Remove from oven and top each muffin with 2 tablespoons custard.

For the custard: you will be using the double boiler method. Therefore, whisk egg yolks, almond milk, and sweetener in a metal bowl. You will then have to slowly mix the melted butter (still warm) in the egg mixture. If not done slowly you will overcook the eggs and not achieve the custard-like texture you desire. You will then need to place the metal boil over a pan of boiling water. The mixture will have to be whisk vigorously and constantly until a thick consistency is achieved. Insert an instant-read thermometer into mixture and ensure that it reads 140 degrees F for about 3 minutes or say about 5 minutes in total (you could also coat the back of a spoon). Remove mixture from over water. You may serve chilled or warmed. To serve it chilled, you would have to prepare before time and refrigerate. Ensure that you whisk before serving.

Nutritional Info (per serving)

- Calories 208

- Fat 15g – 64%

- Protein 16g – 30%

- Carbs 3g – 5%

- Fiber – 1g

<u>Dairy-Free Irish Cream Frozen Custard</u>

Prep Time: 5 minutes

Cook Time: 20 minutes

Servings: 6

Ingredients

- 14 tablespoons coconut oil organic butter if not dairy sensitive (3/4 cup plus 2 tablespoons)

- 4 tbsp MCT oil (needed to create a smooth ice cream)

- 1/2 cup strong brewed decaf coffee/espresso

- 4 large eggs

- 4 egg yolks

- 2 teaspoon vanilla extract (however, it is best to use natural vanilla beans scraped straight from the pod)

- 1/2 teaspoon almond extract

- 1/4 cup unsweetened cocoa powder

- 2 1/2 teaspoon instant coffee granules

- 1/4 cup Confectioners Swerve or equivalent

- 1/2 teaspoon sea salt (helps to keep ice cream soft)

Directions: blend the coconut oil, MCT oil, eggs, yolks, almond milk/water, vanilla bean seeds (discard the pod), cocoa powder, natural sweetener and salt until very smooth. After mixing, transfer the mixture into your ice cream maker. You may explore other options for creating ice cream without an ice cream maker. When finished, remove from the ice cream maker and store in an airtight container in the freezer.

Nutritional Info (per serving)

- Calories 362

- Fat 38 6g 95%

- Protein 4 3g 4%

- Carbs 0 5g 1%

- Fiber 0g

Snickerdoodle Mini Donuts

Prep Time: 10 minutes

Cook Time: 12 minutes

Servings: 8

Ingredients

- 1 cup Swerve

- 8 large eggs

- 2 tablespoons coconut oil or butter if not dairy sensitive

- 1 cup water steeped in 4 cinnamon tea bags 3/4 cup coconut flour

- 1 teaspoon baking powder

- 1 teaspoon cinnamon

- 1 teaspoon vanilla extract

- 1/2 teaspoon sea salt

GLAZE:

- 1 cup coconut oil soft but not liquid (or butter if not dairy sensitive)

- 1/2 cup cinnamon tea strong brewed 3/4 cup Confectioners Swerve

- 1 teaspoon cinnamon

Directions: preheat the oven to 350 degrees F. In a large bowl, combine the eggs, sweetener and oil.

Steep four tea bags in 1 cup water for about 5 minutes. Cool the tea for a while. After the tea has somewhat cooled, pour in the egg mixture. You will not do this all at once but use a method called tempering. You can add a small amount of the warm mixture into the egg mixture, whisking it in slowly. The aim is to get the egg mixture warmer. After this, you can slowly mix in the egg into the tea. If you do this too fast, you increase the chances of the eggs cooking and the mixture will curdle.

In another bowl, sift in your dry ingredients – the coconut flour, baking powder, cinnamon and salt. Incorporate them well. Then add your wet ingredients. Finally, add the vanilla and mix everything until well combined.

You may choose the type pans to bake your batter in. This is dependent on you. If you use a bread pan, the batter will take 25 -30 minutes to be properly baked. When using a muffin tin, it will only take 12- 15 minutes. Before pouring the mixture, ensure that the pan is well greased. You may use muffin liners or greased sheet to prevent the batter from sticking to the tin.

To know if the batter has been properly cooked, insert a clean toothpick into the center and when you remove the toothpick if it comes out clean, this means it's baked thoroughly. Remove it from the oven and let cool in pans for 10 minutes. As they are cooling, make the glaze by placing all the ingredients in a blender or food processor and combine until smooth. Once the bread donuts are cool, pour about 2 tablespoons of glaze over each piece. NOTE: this glaze will separate if it sits out and gets too hot, puree again until smooth. You may also drizzle or dunk the baked goods into the glaze.

Nutritional Information (per serving)

- Calories 440

- Fat 39g – 79%

- Protein 10g – 9%

- Carbs 13g – 12%

- Fiber 9g

Strawberry Cheesecake Ice Lollies

Prep Time: 3 minutes

Cook Time: 0 minutes

Servings: 4

Ingredients

- 4 ounces cream cheese softened (or coconut cream if dairy sensitive)

- 1/4 cup unsweetened vanilla almond milk

- 4 tablespoons Confectioners Swerve (or equivalent)

- 1 teaspoon strawberry extract

Directions: mix the cream cheese, almond milk and sweetener in a bowl until smooth. Slowly stir in strawberry extract (and Strawberry Kiwi Stur if you wish). Pour mixture into Popsicle molds. Place it in the freezer for a minimum of 2 hours, until firm, and then serve.

Nutritional Information (per serving)

- Calories 103

- Fat 10g – 88%

- Protein 2g – 8%

- Carbs 1g – 4%

- Fiber 0.1g

Keto Vanilla Latte Custard

Prep Time: 4 minutes

Cook Time: 1-3 minutes

Servings: 4

Ingredients

- 1 cup coconut milk full-fat (or heavy cream if not dairy-sensitive)

- 1 tablespoon gelatin grass-fed powdered

- 1 cup strong brewed decaf coffee/espresso (1 cup water steeped with 2 chai tea bags)

- 1/2 cup Confectioners Swerve sweetener or equivalent

- 2 teaspoons natural vanilla extract (however, it is best to use natural vanilla beans scraped straight from the pod)

- 1/8 teaspoon sea salt

Directions: in a medium-sized bowl pour in coconut milk, sift in the gelatin. As you prepare the other ingredients, the gelatin mixture will dissolve into the coconut milk.

Over medium heat, in a saucepan, warm the coffee and also heat milk in the microwave for one minute. Whisk the sweetener into the cool coconut milk gelatin mixture. Stir until well combined. Then pour the hot coconut milk into the gelatin mixture while stirring constantly. Then add the extract and salt. Pour the custard into four 4-ounce serving cups. To make the custard set, refrigerate for at least an hour. Best served at room temperature but can be served cold.

Nutritional Information (per serving)

- Calories 105

- Fat 9g – 77%

- Protein 4g – 15%

- Carbs 2g – 8%

- Fiber 0g

Strawberries and Cream Shake

Prep Time: 5 minutes

Cook Time: 0 minutes

Servings: 4

Ingredients

- 8 ounces cream cheese packaged

- 1 1/4 cups unsweetened almond milk (unflavored or vanilla) (hemp milk if nut-free)

- 1/4 cup Confectioners Swerve style sweetener or equivalent

- 1 teaspoon natural vanilla extract (however, it is best to use natural vanilla beans scraped straight from the pod)

- 1 teaspoon strawberry extract

- 1 cup crushed ice

- Healthy Add-Ins (optional):

- 1 tablespoon aloe vera juice pure

- 1 tablespoon l-glutamine powder

Directions: blend all ingredients until the desired consistency is reached.

Nutritional Info (per serving)

Calories 200

Fat 19g – 86%

Protein 4g – 9%

Carbs 2g – 5%

Fiber 0.2g

Supplementing Your Keto Lifestyle

It has been emphasized throughout this guide that there are numerous benefits that one can experience when following a low-carb diet. These benefits can be increased when using a variety of ketogenic products that supplement the diet. Some of these products include:

Ketogenic shake and soup: these are meal replacement products that can be even used as a snack. These may be best to consume before a workout. They include quite a number of fat (on average 14 grams of fat) and up to 20 grams of protein). Note that you need to read labels carefully as you may be consuming more proteins than fat. You should also calculate these amounts in the overall macronutrients you should consume in a day. They may also contain MCT which is great for your keto diet.

MCT oil and MCT powder: this product contains high levels of medium-chain triglycerides. They may be sold in either oil or powder forms which makes it easy to be used in meal preparation. So, you could add MCT in your shakes or when preparing your meals. These are of high quality and therefore, they will be sold in concentrated forms.

Exogenous ketone salts: for temporarily increasing the circulation of these ketones in your body, the ketone salts will make ketones available for use as an additional energy source.

Whey: is a great source of protein and can be used in many meals, especially in the creation of shakes (note the shake recipes provided in this chapter – you may add whey even if not listed as an ingredient) You may also add it to your yogurt so as to increase your daily protein intake.

Creatine: is a natural substance that can be found in muscle cells, but you can take it as a supplement. This helps to improve your performance when working out. It also helps to increase muscle mass and strength.

Keto-friendly Snacks

Though snacking is not encouraged and following the keto diet will allow you to feel satiated most of the time, if you ever do begin to feel hungry throughout the day, make sure to have some keto-friendly snacks on hand. These feelings of hunger are normally experienced by those who are just beginning a ketogenic diet because your body needs time to adjust to the changes in energy consumption. Snacking means that you should use healthy options and so, you have to choose options that will not kick you out of the state of ketosis. Let's group these snacks into two groups. You will have the ready-made options (be honest, sometimes you just do not have the time) and, of course, those snacks that are homemade.

Here are some snacks that you can just grab on the go:

- Iced coffee

- Avocado (can be eaten as is or you can add some salt and pepper)

- Kale chips

- Sardines (though they can be a bit stink, they are rich in fats and other nutrients – just ensure to have some mints on hand)

- Low carb bars

- Olives

- Cherry tomatoes (these have carbs so limit your intake)

- Cheese (Laughing Cow Cheese is a good brand)

- Pepperoni slices (can be highly processed so limit your intake of this food)

- Macadamia nuts

- String Cheese (avoid the fat-free version or those with fillers; ensure that this is made from natural cheese)

- Nut butters are from nuts such as pistachios, peanuts, cashews, almonds, walnuts, etc. (choose those that are natural – no vegetable oil or sugar added.

- Cocoa nibs (not to be confused with chocolate chips that have added sugar; these are crushed cocoa beans that have an intense chocolate flavor with fewer carbs.

- Popsicle (sugar-free)

- Sugar-free Jell-O

- Pork rinds,

- Beef jerky (choose a brand that has low to no carbs)

- Dark chocolate (80% or over; it can be sweetened with stevia or monk fruit)

- Seaweed snacks (examine the ingredients on the package; you should aim to avoid snacks that contain toxic oils or added flavors)

- Fruits such as raspberries, strawberries, blackberries and blueberries

- Keto coffee (this will be coffee that is made without sugars and with full fat cream)

If you have the time and you can prepare your snacks at home. There are a variety of wonderful options that you can choose from. Some of these on the list can be bought, but to ensure that they are not loaded with carbs or hidden sugars, it's best you prepare them at home. You may include some of those items listed above in your homemade snack recipes. Try some:

- Cheeps dips or fondues

- Salads

- Keto smoothie

- Bone broth (you can prepare before time and add fresh herbs before serving)

- Chocolate mousse

- Lettuce wraps

- Cauliflower ice-cream

- Keto pate (make a spread with meat and cream cheese)

- Flaxseed crackers

- Bacon or any keto-friendly food wrapped in bacon

- Pizza with a crust made from cauliflower

- Cold cuts of meat (ham, salami, etc.)

- Boiled Eggs

- Cucumber

- Celery sticks (can be used for your keto-friendly homemade dips)

- Veggie sticks (cut up your favorite vegetables such as zucchini)

There are certain types or brands of foods that we like to enjoy. You can eat them while on the keto diet, only if the ingredients or the way in which they are being prepared aligns with the key rules of the diet. These food include tuna from the can, deli or cold meat (sliced ham, salami, chicken, turkey breast, etc.) and even devilled eggs.

The list of snacks can be extensive and, of course, could not be captured above. So, here are some do's and don'ts for snacking.

Do's:

1. Prepare your own snacks. Yes, it can be time-consuming but consider the fact that you will know exactly what ingredients are used and will be able to judge its appropriateness for your diet plan.

2. Stick to the daily recommended macronutrients. Do not just snack away, forgetting that you have a limit to what you can consume. Snacking healthily does not mean snacking indefinitely.

3. When trying a new snack, even if it is on the list, do your self-testing – test to see how consuming that snack affected the glucose levels in your blood (you may view information on self-testing in chapter three). If it provides a spike in your blood sugar or insulin level, then avoid that snack.

Don'ts

1. Though snacking is accepted with the Keto diet, it is best that you try not to get that hungry to the point of wanting snacks. If you are eating the right ratio of fat: protein: carbs, then you will feel full for longer and will not have the urge to snack.

2. If your schedule does not allow for full meals at all times (even though you should be planning ahead and prepackaging your meals), you may need to have snacks on hand. This will lessen the urge to buy snacks or foods that may not be a part of the diet. Step away from the cream cheese bagel!

3. Have prepackaged snacks without checking the labels. The labels will list the macronutrients. If these are and/or the ingredients are not suitable for a keto diet, then do not consume.

Common Items Used to make Low Carb Weekly Meals Plans easy to use and Versatile

If you feel as if staying on a ketone diet is difficult and food preparation is time-consuming. Just keep the following list as a guide in your kitchen or when grocery shopping so that you can stay on track:

- Have some mayonnaise on hand. Not the fat-free version though. Remember what we discussed above about the fat-free or diet foods – they are loaded with sugars. You can use mayonnaise instead of cream cheese or sour cream.

- Avocados are seasonal and may not be available all year round for some of us, but they can be used in meals to add texture and fat.

- Dairy products. Cheese is optional but if you wish to have lower carb intake, try vegan cheese instead. Also, instead of yogurt, you can use coconut milk yogurt (unsweetened).

- Coconut cream or heavy cream can be used interchangeably.

- Coconut products such as coconut milk or cream (no sugar added) and coconut oil are great in any meal plan.

- Instead of coconut oil, you can also use butter.

- To replace your normal flour that is rich in carbohydrates, use almond or coconut flour instead. However, note that for every cup of almond flour used in a recipe, you can substitute with a ¼ cup of coconut flour.

- If you wish not to consume eggs, you can substitute this with soaked chia or flax seeds.

- Nuts (peanuts, pecans, pistachios, etc.) Nuts can also be substituted in recipes with pumpkin seeds, chia, flax, or even sunflower seeds.

- Nut or seed butters or tahini (made from toasted ground hulled sesame which can be used as a condiment).

- Shellfish or other types of seafood.

CHAPTER SIX – KETO AND EXERCISE

Throughout this guide, you have been getting hints that exercise is crucial to the success of a keto diet. In fact, exercise and a proper dietary plan go hand in hand to ensure your weight loss success. Exercise in a keto diet will see you enhancing your weight loss while building necessary muscle. Most importantly, even though the keto diet provides you with increased energy, coupled with exercise, your energy levels will skyrocket – allowing you to do more throughout your day. How about improving your cardiovascular health, strengthening your bones or even improving your mental health? These are benefits that you will enjoy.

We have already identified that the key to weight loss on this diet is not due to simply cutting calories. You will have to eat the right percentage of macronutrients to see a reduction in your weight. Also, you do not need to have extensive and strenuous exercise sessions along with the keto diet for you to see the results you need. As discussed before in chapter four, working out when you are just beginning the keto diet can help you to alleviate some of the side effects experienced with "keto flu."

Types of Exercise

Just as with any form of diet and exercise plan, there are variations. Therefore, the types of exercises that are best for you to do depends on your own needs. Also, how you exercise will also affect your nutritional needs (note the different types of keto diet, as discussed in chapter one). There are four types of exercise that are great to do while your body is in ketosis:

1. Cardio - Also known as aerobic exercise such as walking, jogging, swimming skipping are low-intensity exercises that you will do over a shorter period of time. These are exercises that increase your ability to burn fat.

2. Weightlifting – Also known as anaerobic exercise. These are exercises that you do for a shorter period of time. They help you to burn carbs as well as build muscles. Muscles building can also be beneficial to your weight loss plan as you are able to burn more carbs even in a state of rest.

3. Stretches – These are exercises that will help you in improving your flexibility. Exercises such as yoga help to improve your soft tissue as well as increase your range of motion over time if practiced consistently.

4. Stability Exercises – With these exercises you aim to strengthen your core and improve your balance. When done properly and consistently, you will see improvements in balance and body control. In addition, they help to support the alignment of your body.

So, if you are seeking to help your body use fat as an energy source, it is best that you do low to moderate-intensity workouts. High-intensity workouts are best in using the glucose consumed or stored in our bodies. You will find it more difficult in completing high-intensity workout initially as your body is using fats for energy and not carbs. If not monitored properly, you may have adverse effects with these types of exercises while on the keto diet.

However, to alleviate such problems, you may need to use a modified version of the diet. Hence, the targeted ketogenic diet (TKD). This diet is for persons who wish to perform anaerobic exercises well while following the diet plan.

TKD

Note that we discussed the difference in this diet before, but to reiterate, the diet allows those who wish to work out to build muscles through strength training to still use the keto diet without negative effects. The idea of this diet is to allow persons to consume carbs when necessary in the right quantities. Remember that the keto diet reduces the number of carbs that one should consume, but energy from carbs is needed for high-intensity workouts.

You will need to determine how much carb is ideal for you to consume to support this lifestyle and which matches your health goal. To do so, you will need to use a ketogenic calculator. You will then be able to, in general, determine the macronutrients that are needed to support your weight loss, then you could have a specific idea of the carbs you should consume to balance your work out.

In a normal keto diet, the recommended amount of carbs which one should eat is between 20 to 50 grams (dependent on your current weight). Some of this will be consumed closer to the time of workout (about 30 minutes prior) and also about 39 minutes after your workout. The best types of carbs to eat are those that are fast-acting. You can get those from fruits, which will provide your body with the necessary glucose so that you can have a sustained high-intensity workout and also during the period of recovery afterward. You will need to consume the standard ratio of ketosis before and after your workout.

Why 30 minutes? In consuming glucose, you are at risk of your body coming out of the state of ketosis because you have given it sugar to burn and not fats. The high-intensity workout will allow you to burn the carbs quickly.

So, there are two main things you should remember before starting this adaptation of the keto diet:

1. Ensure that you have been following the standard keto diet for several weeks and you are in the phase of ketosis or fat adaptation. When in this state for so long, you will be able to slip in and out of ketosis at a much faster rate.

2. You should not have any stores of glycogen. If you do, then when you eat the carbs, the glucose will stay in your blood instead of being stored in your muscles. You need the glucose in your muscles so that you can sustain an effective workout plan. If the glucose stays in your blood, you will no longer be in a state of ketosis.

CKD

For the other types of workout, you can just simply follow a normal keto diet plan. Bodybuilders or athletes will require even more carbs and so, it is best that they use a Cyclical Ketogenic Diet (CKD). On this diet, they will have to increase their carb intake, but this will be balanced by the increased physical activity they take part in and the muscle mass they build. However, this diet is recommended for those who are far advanced in the keto diet.

When implementing the keto diet to a hectic workout routine, it requires that for one to two days, you consume mostly foods that are low in fat but are high in carbohydrates. For the other five to six days of the week, you will follow your standard keto diet. This is necessary to ensure that you use insulin (and other anabolic hormones) to help you to gain the desire muscle mass and to have the necessary glycogen storage to be able to lift weights effectively. You will definitely be removing yourself from the state of ketosis so that you are able to get the optimal results for your training sessions. However, you will still be able to reach your health goals.

Your body needs to use anabolic hormones to help you build muscles (that's why they are also called growth hormones) and burn off fat. For a bodybuilder, this helps them to build the physique that they require.

Phases in CKD

There are two phases of this diet: the standard keto diet and the carb-loading phase. For the former, you will typically have a macronutrients list that states that for five to six days you consume:

- 65-75% fat,

- 5 – 10% carbohydrates,

- and the remaining 15-25% in protein.

You are able to get these macronutrients by consuming foods such as eggs, nuts, butter, coconut oil or olive oil, fatty meats and MCT oil (made from real coconuts).

In this phase, your aim is to keep your insulin levels low, prevent fat gain through the decrease in your glycogen source and increase the levels of growth hormones in your body. For this phase, there is no need to consume carbs after you have worked out. It is believed that consuming carbohydrates here will reverse the effects of increasing growth hormone levels in the body.

In phase two, your carb-loading phase, you are required to consume more carbohydrates for the remaining days of the week (one to two days). On these days your macronutrients should look somewhat like this:

- 5-10 percent fats,

- 15 – 20 percent protein,

- and a whopping 70 percent of your foods should be carbs

On these days, you aim to consume less fat so that your body will burn more glucose for energy instead of fat stored. Other than gaining muscles, there are other benefits to this carb-loading phase. Two such benefits are for you to invigorate your thyroid as well as to restore your adrenals.

Even though increased carb consumption is needed in this phase, these should come from healthy foods. So, even though sweets and donuts contain carbohydrates, these should not be the source of the 70% you need on that day. You will need to avoid simple carbs (empty calories) such as these. Consuming them can lead to inflammation and an unhealthy spike in your blood sugar and insulin levels.

So, what foods should you eat? You need to eat foods that contain complex carbs which takes longer for your body to digest and thus, no sugar spikes. They are called complex carbs because they comprise a long complex make up od sugar molecules bound together. In comparison to simple carbohydrates, they are a greater source of vitamins, minerals and even fiber. So, instead of that soda or white bread, try some sweet potatoes, quinoa, beets, yam, couscous, oatmeal and 100% whole wheat pasta or bread.

After your carb load phase, you will need to get your body back into the state of ketosis. You can only do so the same way that you started the process – reducing the glycogen storage in your body which you had built up while you were eating the extra carbs on those days. When you have done so, your body will go back to burning fats again.

There are some tried and proven ways in which you can help your body to go back into the state of ketosis over a three-day period. These include:

1. One the first day you fast. Intermittent fasting by not eating until dinner time will allow you to start depleting those glycogen stores. Your dinner will consist of a regular keto meal — fewer carbohydrates and more fats, with a moderate amount of proteins. In fact, doing intermittent fasting throughout your diet is very helpful. You will need to set up a time period in which you fast and times when you will consume keto-friendly meals. It may help the body to be or have a more flexible metabolic rate This will mean that your body will be able to speed up the amount of time it takes to readjust to burning ketones instead of fat for fuel.

2. Increase the intensity of your weightlifting. For this activity, your body will need lots of glycogen. So, weightlifting will help you to use that extra amount in your body. Even though you will continue to follow the standard keto diet, when lifting weights on this day, do so on an empty stomach. You can also choose to do some HIIT (high-intensity interval training). This workout regime will require you to perform exercises that require a high burst of energy, but you will only rest for a short time in between each.

3. On the third day, as soon as you wake, do some high-intensity exercises before eating.

You will continue to consume your high-fat, low carb diet.

Workout Regime

Now that you have an understanding of TKD and CKD, let's examine a sample of a weekly workout. Remember that you can switch up the workout and do certain aspects on certain days. For example, if on the first day of week one you do lower body workout, then you can switch and do this on the third day. However, this is after some time (probably about a month; you need your body to have a consistent workout before switching it up). Also note that it is important that you warm-up and cool down after each exercise routine, which will include stretches.

CKD workout sample

This is a sample and there are other exercises that you can do to target sections of the body. The amount of weight or the level of resistance is based on your fitness level.

Day one: focus on your lower body. Your lower body workout may consist of squats, leg press and lunges (4 sets of 12 reps for each). You can also include leg curls and calf raises.

Day two: work your upper body. You can include exercises such as bench press (do four sets of 12 reps). You can finish this workout with biceps curls, triceps extensions or pull-ups.

Day three: this is the day you do some HIIT exercises. You can incorporate cycling, rowing and sprinting. To use them in a high-intensity workout you may sprint for 30 seconds and then rest for the same amount of time. This will be done 10 times. After that you will cycle for a minute and then rest for the same amount of time – this is repeated 10 times. Note these can be mixed together to have your own workout. For example, you may do a set of rowing, then move on to do a round of cycling and then continue in such a pattern.

Day four: Do a full-body workout on this day. Some exercises that can target most if not all muscle groups would be deadlifts, clean and press, pull-ups with weights and barbell rows.

Day five: You will rest on this day. You can switch your rest day to suit your schedule. However, rest is very important to any weight loss/exercise plan.

Day six: You can do a HIIT exercise routine on this day or you may even do a high-rep full-body workout.

Day seven: Walk, jog or do some other low-intensity exercise on this day.

Note that there are many other options available and the choice is ultimately yours. It is also important to note that you do not have to exercise. If you choose to you can do cardio, yoga or any mild exercise. Walking to the corner store is an easy choice. As cliché as it may be, taking the stairs instead of the lift may also help.

CHAPTER SEVEN – KETO AND ILLNESSES

Many people will be eager to start the keto diet because of their desire to see the weight loss results that it promises. They may even be just simply desiring a healthier lifestyle. However, it is befitting to use this final chapter to examine how the keto diet may aid in the control of the reduction of epilepsy-related seizures because this was the first application of the diet before its popularity. It is also good to see instances in which the diet is beneficial in treating ailments that are not related to the most anticipated result of weight loss.

Epilepsy

When surgery is not possible to treat cases of refractory epilepsy and epileptic encephalopathies, a ketogenic diet is considered as a treatment option. Studies show that with all types of seizures the ketogenic diet has been able to assist in alleviating the symptoms of epilepsy experienced. However, this does not mean that it is a cure. For, while patients with focal epilepsy may improve, they do not achieve complete freedom from seizures on the keto diet. The effectiveness of the diet to help those with the ailment is not limited to any specific age group, however, research students have shown its efficiency in helping children with epileptic encephalopathies.

For research studies, it is seen that occasionally, children with show a high level of reduction in the seizures they experienced due to the use of the traditional keto diet (remember we discussed the types in a previous chapter) in comparison to when they are adhering to a low glycemic or modified Atkins diet. However, it should be noted that all ketogenic diets should produce the same results.

The level ketosis low when following a low glycemic index diet but the results have been the same as discussed above. Therefore, it may be surmised the level of ketosis is not the determining fact for the diet's success in alleviating symptoms of epilepsy as previously thought.

The supporting evidence that ketosis works is seen in uncontrolled studies and also the results are experienced by both children and adults, compared to eight months (short term use) versus long term traditional use of the keto diet in infantile spasms. It was found that the use of the diet for only eight months in children who become spasm-free appears to be justified, with similar outcomes, recurrence rate, and less growth disturbance than in two years (longer-term), traditional use. Maybe the keto diet is not an ideal first-line therapy for infantile spasms because of the fact that it usually takes longer to be effective compared to other first-line therapies. Given the concern for the adverse developmental impact of ongoing hypsarrhythmia, if initial options of treatment are used, then the diet should be adhered to and results studied for a maximum period of two weeks. If symptoms are ongoing or worsen, then one should switch the type of therapy used.

Evidence in adults

In comparison to evidence of the effectiveness of the keto diet to treat epilepsy is less robust less tested by researchers. Data suggests that only 38% of the consensus group offered dietary therapy to adults. Other diets that are deemed more flexible and more appetizing are seen as more viable options than the traditional KD, such as the modified Atkins diet or low glycemic index diet. These are seen as a more attractive option for adults with problematic epilepsy. In a study where the keto diet was used as a treatment for adults with refractory epilepsy (generalized and focal), 50% of subjects had greater than 50% reduction in seizures and 33% had more than 85% seizure reduction. The diet was tolerable with mild effects such as nausea, vomiting, diarrhea, constipation, and weight loss. In another study conducted with 30 adults (>18 years-of-age, with at least weekly seizures, prior use of at least two anticonvulsants) using a modified Atkins diet, the results showed that 47% had a more than 50% seizure reduction after one and three months on the diet and 33% after six months. The medium-chain triglyceride ketogenic diet and low glycemic index treatments have not been studied systematically in adults.

Most individuals who develop epilepsy will respond to pharmacologic treatment, however, approximately 20%–30% are pharmacoresistent. For this population, KD can be highly efficacious and should be considered early, as further antiepileptic drug trials have low rates of success. Based on the evidence that is reviewed and authors experience, KD should be offered to both children and adults with intractable epilepsy that is not potentially treatable with surgical options.

There is great evidence in the Canadian Journal of Neurological science that supports the idea that the keto diet aids children with myoclonic-atonic epilepsy. Oguni produced findings which stated that the most effective treatment for myoclonic-atonic epilepsy is adhering to a keto diet. It is then thought that is best that this diet is included as an initial treatment of myoclonic-atonic epilepsy instead of a last resort.

Infantile Spasms

Research carried out in an institution that aimed to evaluate the efficacy of the keto diet on children who suffer from infantile spasms presented results that state that there was a 50% improvement in most of the children (two-thirds) and up to 77% of the children benefitted after two years. The data also stated that 23% no longer experienced any spasms within a six-month period within a median of 2.4 months of starting the keto diet. It should also be noted that the findings stated that 62% had shown improvement in their neurodevelopment, 35% had electroencephalogram (EEG) improvement, and 29% were able to reduce concurrent anticonvulsants. Based on these findings, it is recommended that corticosteroids, adrenocorticotrophic hormone (ACTH) and vigabatrin be used as a treatment for infantile spasms.

Other ailments

Other studies have been conducted to try to determine the correlation between a keto diet and other illnesses. Here are a few:

Cancer

In a research with a mouse who was afflicted with malignant glioma, which was aimed at studying the effects of the ketogenic diet on the disease, it was determined that animals that were fed to adhere to the principles of a ketogenic diet showed elevated levels of β- hydroxybutyrate (p=0.0173) and an increased median survival of approximately five days in comparison to others that were fed a normal diet. Of the 11 animals tested, 9 animals who were treated with a combination of a keto diet and radiation, saw their tumor cells diminished below the level of detection (p<0.0001). Analysis of the results could make one determine that a keto diet significantly enhanced the anti-tumor effect of radiation and could be very effective in being used in conjunction with the current standard of care for the treatment of human malignant gliomas. Another study with two children with anaplastic astrocytoma provided results that indicated that the keto diet used as treatment saw a decrease in the tumor's glucose metabolism as assessed by positron emission tomography (PET). With these results, one can conclude that there needs to be further clinical testing to further examination of the ability of the diet to treat cancer patients.

Headache

Having a headache is a common ailment that plague many in this fast-paced world. There has been evidence that a keto diet with medium-chain triglyceride has aided in the reduction of the velocity of cortical spreading depression in rats. In addition, it was noted that even a modified Atkins diet could help patients who are plagued with chronic daily headaches.

Autism

After a six-month period when 30 children (aged 4-10 years) with autism who were placed on a keto diet in a pilot, the results showed that 18 of them (60%) experienced some level of improvement in several parameters on the childhood autism rating scale. Though the results are very preliminary and significant limitation to the study due to the lack of a control group, this is enough to support the idea that further studies are needed. These should be conducted before this therapy should be considered for autism.

For animals tested who had some form of traumatic brain injury, it showed that adhering to the keto diet reduces cortical contusion volumes that correlate well with beta-hydroxybutyrate levels in serum. This suggests that there is a neuroprotective effect of the diet. There is the need to test this on humans before this treatment is considered beneficial and able to treat persons with traumatic brain injuries.

Of all the studies examined above, it can be concluded that even though there are some results showing the possibilities of the keto diet helping to treat other major ailments. But further studies are needed, where other factors are considered before it is considered to be an acceptable treatment.

CONCLUSION

The keto diet is a meal plan that allows your body to produce ketones and then go into a state of ketosis. Ketones are produced when the body uses fat as the source of energy instead of glucose. This is possible because the diet consists of meals that reduce the intake of sugars and carbohydrates, thus depleting the glucose storage in the body. This is the reason why people are able to lose weight and keep it off when following this diet.

However, loss of weight is not the only benefit of following this diet. People are also able to treat ailments such as epilepsy and also prevent certain lifestyle diseases such as Type I and Type II diabetes. Even though there are some side effects that persons may encounter when they just begin the diet, they do not only alleviate them through applying the suggestions discussed in the book, but the permanent advantages far outweigh their temporary effects. The diet is very simple and easy to follow and can fit into your lifestyle.

Exercise is a very beneficial complement to the ketogenic diet. The diet can be adapted to any exercise plan that you have and provides you with the best results when followed well. The aim is to ensure that the glucose that is needed for workouts is present in the body. With the proper planning of food intake and exercise, one would be able to mitigate the side effects – one such is the body shifting from its ketogenic state. Therefore, it is possible to be a weightlifter, an athlete or anyone who desires to incorporate exercise into their keto lifestyle and still reap the rewards of the diet.

After reading this book, you have now a glimpse at the keto diet and have received enough information to aid you in making that decision to note that the diet will benefit your overall health and wellbeing and provide you with the quality of life you deserve. Whether through reading you have been convinced of applying this diet to your daily life or you were determined to do so before, this beginner's guide would have provided you with guidance, tips, tricks and recipes that will allow you to implement it successfully.

The use of the keto diet in your life will extend beyond just weight loss and will help you to develop a better understanding of foods and allow you to be more aware of what you put into your body. If you do not take care of you, then who else will? Start the diet today and reap the benefits for you to live a long and happy life.

Made in the USA
Coppell, TX
18 May 2020